OUT OF THE
Tempest

To Deb
Mae Jean
5-26-05

OUT OF THE Tempest

A True Story of God's Power to Heal a Storm-Tossed Life

Mae Jean Mason

Pleasant W✦rd

© 2005 by Mae Jean Mason. All rights reserved

Pleasant Word (a division of WinePress Publishing, PO Box 428, Enumclaw, WA 98022) functions only as book publisher. As such, the ultimate design, content, editorial accuracy, and views expressed or implied in this work are those of the author.

No part of this publication may be reproduced, stored in a retrieval system or transmitted in any way by any means—electronic, mechanical, photocopy, recording or otherwise—without the prior permission of the copyright holder, except as provided by USA copyright law.

Unless otherwise noted, all Scriptures are taken from the Holy Bible, New International Version, Copyright © 1973, 1978, 1984 by the International Bible Society. Used by permission of Zondervan Publishing House. The "NIV" and "New International Version" trademarks are registered in the United States Patent and Trademark Office by International Bible Society.

Scripture references marked KJV are taken from the King James Version of the Bible.

Scripture references marked NASB are taken from the New American Standard Bible, © 1960, 1963, 1968, 1971, 1972, 1973, 1975, 1977 by The Lockman Foundation. Used by permission.

ISBN 1-4141-0407-3
Library of Congress Catalog Card Number: 2005901208

Dedication

Dedicated to my heavenly Father and all his helpers who supported me through the stormy times and now share in the joy of my renewal.

Table of Contents

Introduction ix

PART I: TORNADO 1
   Chapter 1:   At Death's Door 3
   Chapter 2:   Never the Same 19
   Chapter 3:   Adjustments 39
   Chapter 4:   Threshold 57
   Chapter 5:   Revelations 75

PART II: HURRICANE 95
   Chapter 6:   Storm Clouds 97
   Chapter 7:   The Pit 115
   Chapter 8:   Through New Eyes 135
   Chapter 9:   Third Wave 153
   Chapter 10: Lost Dreams 171

PART III: RECONSTRUCTION 189
   Chapter 11: Starting Over 191
   Chapter 12: Full Potential 209

Introduction

"Everybody Has a Story" is the name of CBS reporter Steve Hartman's series of human-interest news articles. Steve selects a person for each report by blindly tossing a dart at a U.S. map and picking a name from the targeted area's phone book using another random method. Then he asks the person to share his/her personal story. Some turn out to be heartwarming or humorous while others are gut wrenching. Over the years, Steve has proven his theory that every person has a story to tell. The book you hold in your hands is my story. I am an ordinary person who has had some extraordinary life experiences. I share them in the hope that they will encourage, inspire, and challenge you.

The title, Out of the Tempest, has a dual meaning. First, some powerful "storms" battered my life over a period of many years, but they are over now. I am no longer in the tempest; I am out of the tempest. Second, many pearls of insight and understanding have come to me as a result of those tempestuous times. I have gotten a great deal out of them. I am a better, richer person for having gone through such painful trials.

In 1991, I self-published a short autobiography describing the first storm and the resulting triumph over tragedy. Little did I know that an even more devastating storm was brewing and another triumph would follow. In writing this expanded autobiography, I revised the first book and made it Part I of the new book so the reader has the whole story in one volume. Moreover, my perspective on the first storm has changed somewhat, and the revised version reflects that.

Many people have played a part in my life's story in a variety of roles. Some have blessed me tremendously while others have challenged me in painful ways. As you read about my relationships with them, please keep in mind that each one has his/her own story to tell. Their perspectives on my interactions with them might be very different from mine. I can only share my own and a limited understanding of theirs. The names of some people, places, and institutions have been changed to protect their privacy and to prevent any embarrassment this writing might cause them.

My greatest desire is to show you how the Lord has worked in my life. He has given meaning and purpose to seemingly meaningless suffering. Through all my troubles, he has been faithful to protect my faith in him from the flaming darts of the enemy, the devil, as well as saving me from my own ignorance and misconceptions. God has used my trials as teaching tools to help me grow as a person and has gotten me back on track with his plan for my life. May he touch the hearts of all who read this.

Mae Jean Mason

PART I

Tornado

Chapter 1

At Death's Door

The last weekend in April of 1985 would have been memorable even if the unexpected had not happened. During Sunday morning services at our church there were going to be infant and child dedications, and Denny and I were planning to dedicate our three-year-old son Russell to the Lord. We had put it off for some time. Denny took very seriously the commitment we would be making to raise our son in the Lord's ways and thought he needed to deepen his personal relationship with God first. Now, at last, he felt ready.

We had invited our parents, brothers, and sisters to the dedication and then to our home for dinner afterward. If even half of them came, our little house was going to burst at the seams, but we didn't want to leave anyone out. My plans for Saturday included making Sunday's big dinner. So, while Denny and Russell busied themselves around the farm, I drove into Pleasant Creek nine miles away to buy the groceries I needed to make the meal and to run some other errands.

First, I stopped at the church house to prepare my Toddler Sunday School classroom for the next morning's lesson. From there I went to a clothing store to look at summer clothes. We had just enjoyed a week of warm weather with temperatures reaching as high as 80 degrees (unseasonably warm for late April in mid-Michigan), and I needed more cool tops suitable for wearing while working in the raspberry fields. Most of my spare time that spring was spent cutting canes. Finally, I went to the grocery store and then headed home.

Back at the house, I had a hard time fitting any more food in the fridge. The main problem was the four large containers of beefsteak mushrooms we had picked the day before.

"I think we have enough," I told Denny as we topped off the last container.

"But Mae Jean! We hit the mother lode!" he exclaimed with the mocked enthusiasm of a gold prospector. We had never found so many mushrooms in one place. Previously, we had gone mushroom hunting in the woods along the east side of his parents' berry farm. Now we were picking across the road from the farm on the four-acre parcel we had recently purchased.

"But there's no way we can eat all of these, Denny. If we pick any more, we'll just end up throwing them away."

"We'll give 'em to the neighbors," he offered with a grin and went on picking. He was having fun, but I had other work to do.

"I'm quitting," I announced and headed for the road. Denny and Russell reluctantly followed, and together we crossed the highway to the berry farm.

We called three neighbors to offer them some of our mushrooms. One took some, but the other two said they wouldn't eat beefsteaks because they were poisonous. We had eaten them before without getting sick, so we paid no attention to their warnings.

As I stacked the dishes in the fridge on top of each other to open up more space, I decided to cook some of the mushrooms for lunch and serve them with hot dogs. They looked ugly to little Russell, so he ate just a hot dog. Afterward, I stayed in the kitchen to make lasagna for Sunday's dinner as well as a dish-to-pass for the fellowship meal we were going to on Saturday evening. It was our second "Dinner for Eight", an in-home event organized by our church to bring people together for sharing.

As evening approached, I watched out the living room window as Denny and his pint-sized partner dragged the old raspberry canes out of the field with the tractor and rake and pulled them into a pile for burning. It didn't look like they were planning to quit any time soon, which meant I would probably be going to the meal alone. Getting my dish-to-pass from the kitchen, I went down the stairs, out the side door of the garage, and got into the Chevette. I followed the driveway which circled our barn-style house, the garden, and the root cellar until I came to the cane pile. Denny came over with the tractor and added some more canes. Russell was sitting on his lap having the time of his life.

"It's time to go," I told them after Denny turned off the tractor.

"Well," he said hesitantly as he looked back at the field, "there's a lot to do yet, and I really need to get it done. Will you be upset if I don't go?"

"No, it's okay. I understand."

The warm weather was causing the new foliage on the raspberry canes to grow fast, making it increasingly difficult to thin out the spindly and dead ones. We needed to get the field work done as soon as possible. And it was all up to us now. After Denny's father had passed away the fall before, his mother had handed the management of their small berry business over to us. Kathryn didn't think she could enjoy the work anymore without Joe working by her side. Nevertheless, it was hard going to the fellowship meal alone. Because of Denny's emotional and spiritual struggles over the years, he had not gone with me to many get-togethers with our church family or relatives.

There were ten or eleven people gathered for the dinner instead of the usual eight including our pastor, Elden Lee, and his wife. After the meal, we all went into the living room to visit. Soon I noticed I wasn't feeling well. When the ill feeling turned into serious nausea, I went into the bathroom. After a few minutes it subsided a little, so I decided to leave before it got worse again. I retrieved my dish from the kitchen and made an excuse for leaving a little early. When I arrived home, I hurried up the stairs and headed for the bathroom. There I found Denny sitting next to the toilet.

"You too?!" I asked in amazement. He looked the way I felt.

"Yeah. It hit me when we were in the field, so we quit and came in." Then I remembered the neighbors' warnings.

"Do you think it was those mushrooms?" I asked timidly.

"I don't know. Russell didn't eat any, and he seems fine."

Within a few minutes we both started vomiting. All night long we took turns worshipping the porcelain goddess while the other hugged a basin. Sleeping was almost impossible because the nausea was continuous and the vomiting frequent. Even Russell had a hard time sleeping with all the extra commotion in our one-bedroom house. Once, as I sat on the bathroom floor waiting, I heard his little voice coming from the doorway.

"Don't worry, Momma. You'll det it out," he said to reassure me.

At Death's Door

At daybreak, I began to wonder how long this was going to last. As a former medical secretary, I became concerned about the possibility of dehydration. I talked it over with Denny and then called my old boss, Dr. Oren Palmer, whose home number I dialed from memory. He contacted the Poison Control Center and then called me back. He said it probably was mushroom poisoning and advised us to go to Community Hospital in Pleasant Creek for treatment with IV fluids and Pyridoxine (Vitamin B-6). Denny thought we could wait it out at home but agreed to go. Then I called our parents and Pastor Lee to let them know what was happening. It was disappointing to have to postpone Russell's dedication, but worse yet was knowing it would not have been necessary if we had listened to the neighbors' warnings.

Kathryn offered over the phone to take care of Russell while we were in the hospital. My parents arrived before she did, and Dad said he could drive us into town while Mom waited with Russell for Kathryn. We got into Dad's car, basins in hand, and headed for Pleasant Creek. As we drove away from the farm, we had no way of knowing that a tragedy was in the making. Like a tornado, it would rip through our lives and prevent us from returning home. If we had known, I'm sure we would have said a tearful, heart-wrenching goodbye as we left the farm. Instead, we drove away expecting to return in a day or two.

When we arrived at the hospital, we were placed in separate rooms on the first floor. Admitting information was recorded, blood samples were drawn, and IV fluids were started. Then a nurse came into my room with a large syringe containing the Pyridoxine, which was supposed to stop the nausea and vomiting. She administered it through a special connection in the IV line. After several hopeful moments, I realized that it was not making a difference. Soon another nurse brought in a bottle of the Pyridoxine and hooked it up to the IV. But as the day progressed, no relief came. Later Denny called me from his room down the hall. The Pyridoxine was not helping him either.

We called Pastor Lee to ask him to anoint and pray for us. We also called on our friend Dr. Darryl Edwards, a dentist who was a leader in our congregation, and my dad Paul Rittenour, a lay minister in his own congregation in a nearby community. They all came to the hospital, laid hands on each of us, and anointed and prayed for us. This followed the teaching in the Book of James about praying for the sick. We were confident that God would answer our prayers said in faith and we would soon begin to feel better.

Instead, Sunday turned into Monday with no relief. The nurses brought bottle after bottle of fluids and Pyridoxine. We became progressively weaker due to the lack of nourishment and sleep. The nurses brought me a bedside commode and encouraged Denny to use a urinal in order to conserve our energy. A few people came to visit, but it was hard to carry on a conversation with anyone. Kathryn brought Russell to see us, and he bounced onto my bed for a hug.

"Hi, Momma!" he said with a big smile. It was good to see him but hard to enjoy having him there.

The nurses maintained the constant flow of Pyridoxine into our blood streams. Denny asked one of them if there could be any harmful side effects from getting so much of it.

"No, Denny, it's just a vitamin," she assured him. "We can give you as much as we need to. Your body will use what it needs, and the rest will pass through your system."

Despite the large amounts of Pyridoxine, we experienced only slight improvement through Tuesday morning. Shortly after noon, Dr. Palmer came to my room.

"The blood work shows that you and Denny are suffering some kidney and liver damage," he told me. "I think we should transfer both of you to U of M. There may be something more they can do for you there."

It was a little scary to think we needed the expertise of a place like that, but we had to go. I called Kathryn, and she brought Russell right over so we could see him before we left. In the middle of the afternoon, we were put on stretchers and loaded into an ambulance. Kathryn stood at the back holding Russell, and we waved good-bye before the attendant closed the door.

It was a long ride to Ann Arbor, taking about two and a half hours. When we arrived at U of M, we were taken to separate areas of the Emergency Room. A nurse took a blood sample and briefly went over our situation with me. After a long time, a young man in a white coat came over to me and introduced himself as Dr. Richard Lynn. He would be our attending physician during our stay there.

Dr. Lynn asked me a lot of questions about our lifestyle. Neither one of us drank alcohol, smoked, or used drugs. We grew and canned our own vegetables, we bought fruit by the bushel for canning, and I baked our breads and sweets. We were physically active with gardening, farm work, and biking. Denny worked as a forklift driver at a factory in Pleasant Creek and I was a stay-at-home mom, active in our church. We had no preexisting health problems.

"How do you feel now?" he finally asked.

"I still feel really nauseous, but I haven't vomited since we left Community Hospital. I just feel sort of sore and achy."

Who wouldn't, I thought, *after lying in bed for three days doing nothing but throw up?* It was a relief, though, to realize that the vomiting had stopped. Apparently it had not been necessary to go to U of M after all. I made the assumption that we would stay a day or two while we regained our strength and then be sent home.

After Dr. Lynn left, I waited some more until another young man, Dr. Townsend, came in to see me. He was in training and had been assigned to assist in my care. Denny was assigned to another doctor in training. It was well after dark before I left the E.R. After having chest and abdominal X-rays done, I was taken to a large ward on the sixth floor. The ward was like a very long, wide room with partition walls along each side forming two-bed cubicles. Each cubicle was divided from the center aisle by curtains hanging from the ceiling, and another curtain divided the cubicle in half. Each patient had visual privacy but could hear much of what was going on throughout the ward. I was taken to a cubicle in the middle of the ward where I settled in for the night.

My recollections from the next several days are limited. What I remember most is the overwhelming feeling that my life was slipping away. The sore, achy feeling became a severe, unrelenting pain. My strength dwindled until I could no longer assist the nurses in getting me onto the bedside commode. My vision became blurry and my hearing muffled. Everything seemed to be fading away.

Several isolated incidents from those days stand out in my mind. Once, I heard Dr. Townsend's voice in the aisle as he spoke with Dr. Lynn. He said something about "massive doses of Pyridoxine", and I wondered just how much we had been given. Another time, I heard Dad's voice coming from the aisle.

"Can we come in?" he asked.

"Yes!" I answered with relief. "Thank God you're here." It was so good to know that I wasn't alone. I knew my parents would watch out for me, which was something I no longer felt capable of doing for myself.

Later, I recall rubbing my forehead. It had gone numb along with the front portion of my scalp. *How strange*, I thought.

On another occasion, I saw Denny's brother-in-law Carl Smith sitting on a chair next to my bed.

"I'm gonna die, Carl! I'm gonna die!" I cried.

"No, Mae," he said soothingly as he rubbed my shoulder. "You're not going to die."

One night I found myself sitting at the edge of the bed looking into the blurry face of a nurse who was sitting on a chair in front of me. She was holding my hands and talking to me.

"Mae! You can't go on like this," she said earnestly. "You need your rest." Well, that was easy for her to say; she wasn't the one who was dying. I wasn't sure if she was pleading with me or scolding me but resolved in my confused mind to stop doing whatever it was that made her say that.

Another night I tried desperately to talk with a different nurse about my imminent death. Since we had no will and Denny was presumably as bad off as I was, I attempted to make provision for Russell by telling her who should be his parents after we were gone.

At some point on Thursday, I watched as a nurse injected a black substance from a large syringe into a tube sticking out of my nose. Someone said it was charcoal. Later, I felt myself begin to vomit, but I was too weak to sit up. A nurse pulled me up into a sitting position.

Another time I saw a little brown teddy bear lying on the bed beside me. I knew it was from my oldest sister and her husband, Pati and Matt Wolfgang, though I couldn't recall seeing them. I tried to pick up the bear, but my hand wasn't working right and I dropped it. The second attempt was successful, and I held the furry bear against my cheek. For some reason it didn't feel right. Sometime later, I saw Matt sitting near me. I didn't have the strength to carry on a conversation but felt I should at least greet him. I attempted to say "hello" and then closed my eyes to take a nap. I was so incredibly tired.

When Dad went to Community Hospital on Monday to visit us, we were both feeling pretty bad, so he didn't stay long. Then he and Mom went together on Tuesday evening to see us. No one had called to tell them of our transfer to U of M during the afternoon. When they found our beds empty, they feared that we had died. They anxiously asked about us at the nurses' station, and Dr. Palmer was paged. He came to the station and told my parents that the transfer was just a precaution. Our prognosis was good.

But on Wednesday evening they received two unsettling phone calls. The first was from one of our doctors at U of M. He said my speech and movements were becoming very lethargic and I might slip into a coma. The other call was from Denny's brother-in-law Carl. Denny's sister Holly and her family lived in Rochester and so were closer to Ann Arbor than any other relatives. Carl came to see us after work on Wednesday and was stunned by what he found. Denny and I were losing ground quickly, and we both told him we were dying. We told him who we wanted Russell to live with, what should be done with our four acres, and where some valuables were hidden in our house. Carl called my parents and Kathryn as soon as he got home.

Mom and Dad drove to Ann Arbor on Thursday morning to be with us. When Dad asked me if they could come into my cubicle, my answer came slowly and with much difficulty. Throughout the day as they sat with us, we begged them to hold our hands constantly, fearing we would slip away if they let go for even a moment. Our speech was slow and our tongues swollen. Chest X-rays showed that our lungs were filling up with fluids. We were in a lot of pain but were also complaining of feeling very hot.

On Thursday evening, tubes were put into our stomachs through our noses so that liquid activated charcoal could be administered. It was hoped that it would absorb some of the excess Pyridoxine. Denny was sitting on a bedside commode when he was given the charcoal. His older brother John from Bay City was there with him. A young nurse named Gina injected the charcoal into his tube, and within seconds he violently through it back up, making quite a mess for Gina to clean up. In spite of how sick he was, Denny exchanged a few words and a grin with John when she left about how pretty she was.

When I was given the charcoal, I was able to keep it down until about 3:00 a.m. Friday. Because I was lying down when it came up and was too weak to help myself, I aspirated some of it. My lungs were suctioned to get the charcoal out, but they didn't get it all and pneumonia began to develop.

My parents stayed with us continuously, and Carl came each evening, calling Kathryn afterward to keep her informed. On Saturday morning, Pati and Matt took Mom and Dad's place so they could go home for a while. Pati and Matt planned to stay until their return on Sunday. During the night, Pati spent most of her time with Denny who begged her to rub his aching back and leg muscles. Each time she checked in on me I seemed to be resting all right.

Late Sunday morning Matt, who had been resting in the lounge at the far end of the ward, relieved Pati. While sitting on a chair near my bed, holding my hand and talking to me, he suddenly saw my chest sink in and knew I had stopped breathing. He quickly left my bedside in search of a nurse. There were none in the ward. He ran to the nurses' station located at the end of the main hall next to the entrance to the ward. When he told everyone there that I had stopped breathing, they didn't believe him. He wasted no time with them but headed down the hall to Denny's room hoping to find a nurse with him.

Gina was just coming out of the room, and Matt told her I wasn't breathing. She too was reluctant to believe him but went with him to my cubicle anyway. As soon as she saw my blue pallor, she yelled an emergency code word several times and started pulmonary resuscitation. A respiratory team was called in to take over the fight to save my life. Matt went to the lounge to wait with Pati, and a nurse joined them.

"Mom and Dad are due back here any time," Pati told her anxiously. "I don't want them walking in on this."

"I'll try to catch them at the elevator," the nurse said. But as she walked through the ward toward the main hall, she saw my mother coming.

When Dad had gotten up that morning after a less-than-restful night, he had had a strange feeling that something was wrong. Not wanting to scare Mom, he had said nothing to her about it but had tried to hurry her along as they packed some extra clothes in a suitcase. Three hours later as they walked down the sixth floor hall, Dad stopped briefly at Denny's room while Mom went on into the ward. To her surprise, a nurse grabbed her firmly by the arm.

"You're Mae's mother, aren't you?" she said.

"Yes," Mom answered.

"Mae's having a problem right now. We're going down to the lounge together. Don't look as we go by Mae's bed." And they hurried to the lounge.

Leaving Mom with Pati and Matt, the nurse started back through the ward in the hope of catching Dad, but she was too late. He was standing in the aisle watching the respiratory team work over my lifeless body. She escorted him to the lounge, too, where my family waited for word of my fate.

At Death's Door

A female patient in a bed near mine became agitated by the crisis. She told people that the same thing was going to happen to her some day. As her anxiety worsened, she began moving frantically through the ward, slapping people and yelling. Hospital Security was called to deal with her. Soon I was transferred to the Intensive Care Unit (ICU) on the tenth floor. My family was given my personal effects and allowed to follow close behind.

I knew something was wrong even before I opened my eyes. My lungs were hurting, I couldn't make them work, and I was fighting for air. My eyes sprang open, and I saw a man standing over me squeezing a bag which was attached to a tube in my throat. *He's breathing for me,* I reasoned. *Otherwise, I wouldn't be conscious right now.* And I relaxed a little. Then, unable to acknowledge the reality of the moment, I became angry. *If this is some sort of precautionary measure, I am really going to be mad.*

There were several people around me, and we were waiting by the elevator. To my right I saw a young nurse with long, flowing brown hair. It was Gina. Her beautiful hair held my attention for a moment until I lost consciousness again.

When I came to, I was in ICU. The tube in my throat was connected to a respirator. A man in a white coat was doing something to my left wrist, and a nurse was working near my right collarbone. My back was hurting terribly, and I wanted to tell them. I couldn't talk, though, because of the tube in my throat, and I had lost all use of my limbs. So I tried to get their attention by rolling my head and shoulders from side to side.

"Don't do that or we'll have to strap you down," the nurse said and went on working. Her words hit me like ice water. I stopped abruptly and stared at her. Could she possibly mean what she said? Didn't she care that I was trying to get her attention?

I suddenly realized that I no longer had a voice in my physical care. I would have to endure any pain they were unaware of and any treatment they decided was necessary. I couldn't ask for, or object to, anything. My last words to my husband, son, and family had been spoken. There would be no final good-byes. I had been inching closer and closer to death's door and now found myself on the threshold. *From here on it's just you and me, Lord*, I thought.

As I endured my physical agony, I stopped paying attention to the people around me and began instead to think back over my life. I had grown up in a poor but loving home with wonderful Christian parents. I had been a scholastic achiever in high school and college. I had married at 20, worked as a medical secretary, given birth at 24, taught Sunday School, lived a good life. As I scanned everything I had ever done, my thoughts kept returning to a revival service in May, 1974, where I had gone to the altar and publicly acknowledged my need for the redemptive work of God's son, Jesus. It was the only thing that really mattered. The rest was incidental.

I prayed for Denny and Russell, placing them in God's hands. I thought of how difficult it would be for my parents to cope with my death. I could almost hear new acquaintances asking them how many children they had, and their response would be, "We have three daughters, but we used to have four." I knew my heart would probably stop soon. Would there be a big pain in my chest? Maybe it would quit when I was unconscious. It really didn't matter. Finally, I tried to occupy myself by thinking of some favorite hymns while I waited to die. It was Sunday, May 5, 1985.

At Death's Door

That evening in her home to the north, Kathryn sat in her swivel rocker holding Russell on her lap and thinking about the latest word from Ann Arbor. Denny and I were both in ICU and I was on a respirator. The outlook was very grim. Having lost her husband just six months before made it all the harder for Kathryn to cope with our tragedy. Russell looked up into his grandmother's face and saw tears running down her cheeks.

"Don't cwy, Damma," he said, putting his little arms around her neck.

At 68 years old, it was a challenge keeping up with an active preschooler, but she was thankful to have him there. His companionship was making this difficult time bearable.

Year: 2005

Dear Mom and Dad,

I can only imagine how hard it was for you to go through that crisis with me 20 years ago. As a parent myself, I know you would have gladly traded places with your suffering child. We cannot stop bad things from happening, but there are some things we can do to prepare for hard times, and you had done them for yourselves and for your children.

First, you did your best to maintain a close relationship with each of us girls. On more than one occasion, Dad, you have acknowledged that you and Mom were not perfect parents while raising us but feel proud that we turned out to be decent, hardworking women. Now my own child is an adult, and I feel the same kind of personal inadequacy and parental pride. The close, supportive relationship you fostered made such a difference in the midst of the storm.

Second, you planted the seeds of faith in me, which others have watered and God has made to grow. I don't know how I would have survived the trials awaiting me without having the foundation of my life laid on the immovable Rock, Jesus. Thank you for choosing to believe in him and for passing your faith on to me. It is a priceless legacy.

With much love,
Mae Jean

Chapter 2

Never the Same

I was not looking for a husband when I met Denny, though I did want to get married some day. At the time, I was busy with my college studies and was looking forward to working in my chosen vocation—executive secretary. It could take me into almost any field, but I leaned toward medical secretarial work. As far as marriage was concerned, I figured the Lord would bring someone to me when the time was right; I didn't need to look for a mate. Denny, on the other hand, desperately wanted to find a wife. He had dated a few girls and found them to be too "shallow". He wanted a companion who would be serious about her commitment to him and would make a good mother for his children.

After high school, Denny had gone to Chicago to attend an electrical trade school. A year later, he returned to Michigan to find a job. He worked at several short-term jobs over the next three years, the last one being at a factory in Utica. After working there for only three weeks, he lost part of the fingers on his left hand in a press accident. Ten months later, his hand well healed, he was having a hard time finding another job. He couldn't afford his own place and so was living with his parents again. He was an unhappy 23-year-old with a damaged hand, no job, no sweetheart and no home to put her in. Then one lonely day he fell to his knees under a cluster of birch trees at the back of the farm and begged God to send him a wife.

Several days later I walked through the front door of his parents' home while he was eating breakfast. I had come with Pati and her first husband Jim who was planning to go scuba diving with Denny. Pati had invited me to go along to fish with her while the guys were diving. She hadn't bothered to mention to Denny that I would be joining them. Denny took an interest in me right away. Later in the day, as Pati and I fished, he kept peeking over the side of the canoe to say "hi".

"Catchin' anything?" he would ask with a boyish grin.

"No, but we might if you would stop swimming under the canoe."

"Oh." But he came back for little chats ever so often just the same.

Soon he was sure I was the answer to his prayer. He had known Pati for a while and thought she was one of the nicest girls he had ever met. He had been unaware, however, that one of her younger sisters was eligible. He knew about Sue, who was already married by then, and 14-year-old Pam.

"But Pati never told me she had a sister in college," he later said. He was overjoyed by the discovery.

We started seeing each other regularly and found that we had a lot in common—our Christian values, our desire to have children, a love for country living, and laughter. Soon we knew we wanted to get married but agreed to wait until after I finished my two-year degree the next spring. In the meantime, Kathryn helped Denny get a job at the factory where she worked in Pleasant Creek. Since we had almost no money for a home, we decided to convert the loft over the garage Denny was building at the farm into a one-bedroom apartment. When we got married in July, 1977, the loft was shelled in but completely bare inside. We moved in anyway—two young lovers anxious to play house. Within weeks I was also employed.

Over the next four years, we worked at our jobs at the factory and doctor's office during the day and worked on the little loft house in our free time. It took a while to finish it, but we didn't mind. At least we were together. When Russell was born in 1981, I quit my job to stay at home with him. Between marriage, mothering, gardening, and sewing, I was very content.

Denny's job at the factory turned out to be a stable one. Nevertheless, he went through many bouts of emotional and spiritual turmoil. I didn't understand why since he seemed to have a good relationship with the Lord and had many of the things he desired in life. I tried to be a supportive wife and prayed for him often, but I wished there was something more I could do for him. Our church attendance was sporadic because his inner struggle made him feel uncomfortable in church services. When Russell turned two, I told Denny I wanted to take him to Sunday School every week for his spiritual nurturing. He gladly let us go but seldom joined us.

Then in the summer of 1984, Denny's personal battle became unbearable. He went to the church house on a Wednesday evening to pray at the altar and "get things right with God". Afterward, he seemed happier and more at peace. Whatever had been burdening him had apparently been resolved, and we began attending services as a family on a regular basis. Soon I started teaching the toddler Sunday School class.

Since we planned to have more children, we needed a bigger home. We thought about converting the garage into living space or building a larger house there on the farm. Neither option was practical, though, since we had no ownership in the land. Denny's name was on the deed as a survivor, but he really didn't own it. We needed to buy some property, preferably something close to the farm so that some day when his parents handed its management over to us we would be within easy driving distance. Fortunately, we were able to buy four acres directly across the road. While we were saving money to build a house, we spent some time clearing saplings and old stumps from the portion where we planned to build.

When Denny's father died unexpectedly in October, 1984, Kathryn was not sure what to do with their berry business. During the winter, she decided to turn it over to us. In the spring, we worked in the raspberry fields and made plans for marketing the berries in the summer. In late April, we took some time off to go mushroom hunting, thus starting the chain of events that had brought us to the Intensive Care Unit of a big university hospital.

When Denny was moved to ICU on Sunday afternoon, he didn't want to go. No one had told him of my arrest or their concern that he would also develop serious respiratory problems. They didn't feel it would help him to know. In years to come, he would not recall his concerns about dying during those first days at U of M. He would, however, remember well the intense pain and heat, the impaired vision and hearing, and the progressive weakness and incoordination. His clearest memory of all would be the pretty nurses, probably because they were a pleasant distraction from his suffering.

Some time after dark on that fateful Sunday, I saw Pastor Lee coming into my room with Dad. He read a psalm from the Bible, prayed for me, and spoke words of encouragement. I tried to concentrate on what he was saying, but I didn't even have enough energy left to do that. Pastor Lee stayed at the hospital until the early morning hours before heading back to Pleasant Creek. Since Pati and Matt needed to go home to work the next day, Mom and Dad remained alone to maintain the vigil.

Monday was a tense day as they watched my monitor show signs of a weakening heart and saw me try to scream from the pain caused by a gentle squeeze to the hand. Dad made several phone calls to keep relatives and friends posted. He also sent a telegram to my other older sister, Sue, and her family in Germany where her husband Dave was stationed in the Army. That day I was aware of only one thing—unbearable heat. A high fever from the pneumonia, combined with the excessive heat sensation I had already been experiencing, made me feel like I was roasting to death from within.

But on Tuesday things changed. The fever started to come down, the terrible pain subsided a little, and I became fully aware of my surroundings again. I took my first good look around the room I had spent the last two days in and counted the wires and tubes attached to my body. There were six: the respirator, a feeding device below my right collarbone, an IV in my right arm for medications, a device for taking arterial blood samples in the left wrist, a catheter for urinary output, and wires to a heart monitor on my chest.

A limited degree of control had returned to my hands. When my parents came into the room, I gestured with my right hand, indicating that I wanted to write something. They got a pen and some paper from a nurse, but I couldn't maintain a good grip on the pen. So the nurse wrote the alphabet on the paper, and I began to point to the letters, spelling out words and sentences.

It was great to be able to "talk" again. I could communicate my physical needs to the nurses and converse with visitors. One of my first questions to Dad was, "What happened when I arrested?" Dad wasn't sure it would help me to know the details, so he explained the circumstances of the arrest in vague, unalarming terms. But my thinking was clear, and I could see that God had spared my life. If Matt had not been with me when I stopped breathing, I would have surely died. I was ebullient and felt a new confidence that I was going to be okay. In the next room, Denny was also feeling a calm inner assurance that God's hand was on him and he would make it.

Although I was feeling pain and heat at very high levels, the surface of my skin had no feeling at all. I was completely numb from head to toe including the inside of my mouth and throat. Internally, many of my organs were not functioning properly. In addition to my lungs, my digestive system was not working normally, causing my abdomen to swell until I looked several months pregnant. Neither Denny nor I were able to control urination and so were catheterized. Our hearts were racing at over 135 beats per minute, and our blood pressure was seriously elevated. We were being given several medications in an attempt to alleviate these problems.

I was happy to learn that Denny did not need a respirator. I wished I could see him and talk to him, but it was not possible. Later in the day, however, when Denny's brother John and his wife Sarah came to see us, Sarah asked if I wanted to dictate a letter to him. It took a long time to write just a few sentences, but Sarah was very patient as I spelled them out one letter at a time. I told Denny I couldn't wait to leave and do things together again; simple pleasures seemed so important now. With Sarah's help, he sent back a short note, telling me that he loved me.

It was hard to be separated as a couple and as a family, especially under such difficult circumstances. We three had done everything together. Since our marriage, Denny and I had only spent two nights apart, those being when I was in the hospital following childbirth. Russell didn't know the meaning of the word "baby-sitter". Denny missed his little buddy terribly. Mom taped a small picture of Russell to the rail of his bed, and his sister Holly brought each of us a framed 5x7 photo of the three of us. We really appreciated those pictures.

Because Denny did not develop serious respiratory problems, he was returned to Level 6 after a couple of days while I remained in ICU. My lung function gradually improved, and after five days my doctor, Annette Bernard, told me she was going to remove the respirator. I was thrilled by the news and spelled out to my parents that my first spoken words were going to be "Praise the Lord!". But when the respirator tube was pulled out, I couldn't make a sound. Dr. Bernard explained that my vocal cords were swollen. It would be several days before I could talk again. She also told me the cause of our problems.

"The massive amounts of Pyridoxine you received has caused extensive nerve damage. We can't say for sure how long it will take for your nerves to heal. The only thing we have to compare it to are research studies on the effects of large doses of Vitamin B-6 done on dogs and cats. Based on that, we think your nerves will heal in six weeks to three months."

It sounded like such a long time, but I knew how fortunate we were to even be alive. Life would be so sweet when this was over and we went back to the farm to live and work and play.

I remained in ICU for several more days and had a steady flow of people to keep me occupied. Many family members came, including Kathryn who left Russell with Pati and Matt for a day so she could come to Ann Arbor. Many of our church friends came as well as my former college roommates. My parents told me that Dr. Palmer had been there once when I was asleep, and I was sorry I had missed him. Several specialists also came in to check specific aspects of my condition. An EMG and an EEG were done, and a portable X-ray machine was brought in daily to look at my lungs. Drs. Lynn and Townsend came up from Level 6 to see how I was doing, sometimes bringing along the medical students who made rounds with them each day.

Our church friends told me about a special service which had been held on the Sunday I arrested. No evening service had been planned for that day because many church regulars were involved in a community hunger walk in the afternoon. But when word of our transfer to ICU reached our friends, more than thirty people gathered at the church house to pray for us. A man and a woman served as our stand-ins while the others laid hands on them and prayed for us. Their concern deeply touched my heart. I was told of other churches we had never attended that were interceding for us as well. Two pastors from the Ann Arbor area came to visit, and friends were calling friends across the country to place our names on prayer lists. It was overwhelming.

Although I was feeling spiritually high, my physical low persisted. The pain was still significant, and air conditioning gave me little relief from the heat. My ability to move my limbs was limited, so a physical therapist did range-of-motion exercises on me each day to keep my joints from getting stiff. I had nightmares about death and sometimes woke up with a frightening spinning sensation in my head. Dealing with the pneumonia was harder without the respirator. With it, the nurses could easily suction my lungs through the tube, but without it I had to cough up the mucus on my own. Since I had no feeling in my mouth and throat, I couldn't locate the mucus to spit it out. Nurses and family members had to suction it from my mouth.

After nine days in ICU, I was transferred back to Level 6. Because of my need for suctioning whenever I coughed, my parents set up a schedule of round-the-clock visitors for me. Two people came at a time. They took turns sitting with me over a 24-hour period until the next two people came. I was

Never the Same

surprised by some of the aunts, uncles, cousins, and friends who volunteered.

Both Denny and I began having strange physical sensations and hallucinations that were caused primarily by the nerve damage. We felt at times like we were floating around the room or falling into a hole in the bed. One night I involuntarily gasped for air every fourth or fifth breath, had saliva pouring out of my mouth, and felt like I had chips of something on my tongue.

As the days passed, Denny and I grew increasingly anxious to see each other, so the nurses brought him to my room. Because of his pain sensitivity, they had to pick him up with a sheet to put him into a padded, reclining wheelchair for the visit. We had not seen each other since the ambulance ride, and we looked very different. We were pale and had a frightened, wide-eyed look. Denny's weight had dropped from 168 pounds to 134. Mine had gone from 102 to just 80 pounds. We struggled to understand why all of this was happening to us and wondered how long we would be in the hospital. After just a few minutes, he had to leave because he couldn't tolerate being in the padded chair for very long.

We also grew anxious to see Russell. Denny wanted his mother to bring him to the hospital, but I didn't feel ready yet because of the extra strain on me from the pneumonia. One day when the nurses transported me by padded wheelchair to Denny's room, I found him crying.

"My boy! I miss my boy!" he sobbed. I didn't know what to say.

Then on Kathryn's next visit she brought Russell to see us. She didn't let him come into my room at first but left him in the hall with my mother.

"I know you didn't want me to bring Russell yet," she said, "but I did it anyway. He's out in the hall with Mary. Mae, Russell is starting to talk about his mommy and daddy in the past. Even though I keep telling him you're in a hospital, he thinks you're dead. He needs to see you."

Knowing he was just outside the door, I agreed to let her bring him in. I had not seen him in three weeks, and already he had changed. He had gotten his first barber haircut (I had always cut his hair) and was wearing some new clothes Grandma had bought for him. He even looked taller. Kathryn set him on the bed next to me. I tried to talk to him, but he didn't say anything back. He seemed uneasy and a little stunned. After a few minutes, she took him down the hall to see Denny. When Russell was put on the bed next to him, Denny joked with him and tried to tickle him. Slowly Russell warmed up and started smiling and talking with his daddy.

As we talked with Kathryn about Russell's stay with her, we discovered that she was doing some things that troubled us. She was giving him too many sweets and other unhealthful foods and was lax on discipline. She was being a typical grandmother, and if our hospitalization had been a short one, we would have overlooked it. But she was also not willing to take him to church for us even though Denny begged her to.

Because of the intensity of our suffering, it was hard to maintain a balanced perspective. We had lost control over most things and wanted desperately to maintain control over Russell's care. We discussed the possibility of having him live with Pati and Matt for the remainder of our hospital stay, but the idea made Kathryn upset. It called into question her ability as his caregiver. As a loving grandmother, she was doing her best to take good care of him while under great stress. She became angry with us and made her feelings known. We didn't know what to do, so I asked my mother for advice.

"Even though things aren't exactly the way you want them for Russell," she said, "I think it would be best for him to stay in one place and not be moved around. He needs the stability right now." Her advice made sense, and we chose not to move him.

One day Dr. Palmer came to see me again, and this time I was awake. His brief visit was cordial but strained. I didn't know what to say under the circumstances. I think he felt the same way. After all, he was the one who had given us the Pyridoxine and caused our suffering. I didn't feel angry with him, just hurt and confused.

Days passed, and our conditions improved slightly. By late May, our vision and hearing problems were gone, my pneumonia had cleared, and my 24-hour visitor schedule had been dropped. In place of the IVs, we were being fed and medicated through tubes in our noses. But we remained bedridden, unable to do anything for ourselves. We continued to endure the pain and heat, and our internal problems persisted. With little strength and coordination, we were going to need a lot of therapy in the coming weeks. We were already being visited daily by a physical therapist for range-of-motion exercises and a speech therapist who worked on speech problems caused by the numbness of our mouths and lips. For more extensive therapy, our doctors arranged for our transfer to the Rehabilitation Unit on the eight floor.

We had spent a long time on Level 6. The person we were going to miss the most was Gina. She had been good to both of us but especially to Denny, giving him extra TLC many times when he needed it. On May 31, we said our good-byes and were taken to Eight West Rehab.

After being in separate rooms for a month, our new doctors put us together in the hope that it would help us emotionally. But as we lay side by side in our hospital beds, each one had to endure his own physical torment plus the added heartache of watching the other one go through the same thing. People often say it is harder to be the one standing helplessly by a loved one's bedside than to be the one in pain. We were doing both at the same time. After about a week, the staff saw that being together was making things worse for us, not better, and moved Denny to another room.

We soon learned from the staff that our case was a first in their unit. They had dealt with patients before who had suffered nerve damage, but none had completely lost the sense of touch. And they had never worked with a married couple where both people had the same ailment. Sometimes our unique case made it hard for them to know how to help us.

During our first week there, a Rehab social worker came to our room to do an emotional evaluation. She was kind and compassionate but unable to comprehend what we were going through. At one point, she said we needed to consider how our physical problems were affecting our sexual relationship. Of course we missed being intimate, but we also missed more basic activities like walking, eating, and going to the bathroom independently. Our main "desire" was to be free of pain. Denny's patience was at an all-time low, and he became angry with her inability to understand. When she finally asked him to describe his condition for her, he blew up.

"You want to know what it's like?! It's pure hell!" he snapped.

Overall, the staff members worked hard to make their patients as comfortable as possible. Each one was assigned a primary nurse and an associate nurse to manage his/her care. My primary was Lisa, a Rehab veteran, and my associate was Susie, a recent graduate still developing her patience. Denny's primary was bouncy Kelly who sang Mary Poppins songs to him, and his associate was Kathy, a recent graduate with the skill of a pro.

The staff wore street clothes instead of uniforms, and patients were encouraged to wear their own clothes instead of hospital gowns as soon as they were able. There was a day room where patients could eat together, spend time with visitors, work on puzzles, or play board games. It all helped to make Rehab feel less like a hospital. The other patients were going through traumatic times just as we were. Their afflictions included broken backs and necks, diseases, strokes, and attack injuries. One teenage girl had been shot in the neck by her boyfriend and was completely paralyzed, dependent on a ventilator.

To strengthen our muscles and improve our coordination, we began receiving physical and occupational therapy twice daily, five days a week, but progress was very slow. The speech therapist worked with us on making clear sounds without relying on the sense of touch. My speech problems were made worse by the braces on my teeth, so they were removed. The severe pain and heat sensation improved only slightly, and muscle spasms presented a new challenge. Sometimes the nurses had to tie my ankles to the bed with strips of gauze in order to control my jumpy legs. Denny's spastic arms accidentally jerked out his feeding tube on several occasions.

The sense of touch continued to be absent. Fortunately, Denny did regain partial feeling in his mouth and throat and began to eat a little. One day the feeling in my mouth, throat, and on my face returned, and I was thrilled. I asked my doctor for something to eat, but he said "no"—not until a special test could be done to see if the feeling in my throat was adequate for proper swallowing. He would only allow me to have ice chips.

"What about popcicles then?" I pleaded.

"Okay," he smiled. "You can have popcicles." Lisa, my primary nurse, was impressed.

"You're going to let her have flavor?!" she teased.

It was good enough for me. Lisa put a box of popcicles in the day room refrigerator, and my visitors fed them to me in small pieces. I cherished the sensation on my face as well. A night nurse, who often laid his hand on my arm or shoulder while talking to me, gladly put it on my cheek so I could feel it. To my great dismay, the sensation only lasted a few days. The test on my throat had not yet been done, and I had not eaten anything. The doctor told me not to be discouraged, though. The feeling would probably come and go a few times before it became permanent. So I remained hopeful.

The functioning of our internal organs gradually returned to near normal. The first time I was able to release my urine was in the middle of the night, and I wet the bed. The nurses were excited with me that I was getting some control back, though I never would have thought beforehand that wetting the bed was something to get excited about.

Denny and I continued to receive tremendous support from our families and friends. Mom and Dad came to see us once or twice a week, and Kathryn brought Russell about once a week. Other family members, friends from church, and some of Denny's co-workers at the factory visited as often as they could. On June 15, my 28th birthday, seven women from our congregation and the women's Bible study I attended came with all the fixings for a birthday party. Some of my family was there, too. It was a touching gesture, but it was an emotionally difficult experience under the circumstances.

The month of July brought more substantial physical improvements. The sensation of being too hot all the time finally went away, and the pain and spasms lessened. Therapy was helping to strengthen our muscles and improve our coordination. Despite still having partial numbness in his mouth, Denny was able to eat enough solid food to have his feeding tube removed. I regained the feeling in my throat, the special test was done, and I was allowed to begin eating pureed foods.

Except for limited return of feeling in our throats and Denny's mouth, we still had no sense of touch. We learned from our doctors how this was affecting our balance and coordination. The sense of touch lets a person know where his body is in space so he can keep himself "lined up" with his shoulders, hips, and knees all in a straight line when standing. It gives him the ability to move without watching each body part to be sure it is responding properly to the brain's commands. The doctors referred to this ability as "position sense" or "proprioception".

Without it, we had to compensate with our eyesight and watch every move we made in order to perform even simple tasks. One day in occupational therapy, I was putting pieces of wood that had holes in the middle of them on a peg board propped up on a table. The goal was to reach the highest row of pegs. When I successfully reached a higher row than the day before, I turned toward my therapist and smiled triumphantly only to have my arm drop to the table with a painful thud. When I had taken my eyes off my arm and hand, I had lost control of them.

Over time, it became evident that our recovery was going to take a long time. Our internal organs were functioning better and our muscle strength was increasing, but there was no more return of the sense of touch. Improvements in coordination came through learning how to use our eyesight to guide our bodies through basic tasks such as sitting up at the edge of the bed, brushing our teeth, and turning the pages of a book. Walking was impossible because it required more visual and mental concentration than we were capable of. When EMG's showed no sign of the return of our sensory nerves, our prognosis for full recovery was changed to 12-18 months, if at all. One of our Rehab doctors sat down with us individually and discussed our future.

"You need to realize that you'll probably never walk again," he told me. "You will both need help 24 hours a day for the rest of your lives. Chances are you won't regain the ability to take care of your basic needs like bathing and making meals, and you won't be able to take care of Russell by yourselves."

It was beginning to look that way, but I wasn't ready to give up hope for a full recovery. I reminded him that the feeling had come back in my mouth and on my face once. I pointed out that even if the sense of touch didn't come back through natural healing, I knew the Lord could heal us instantly at any time. But in the back of my mind I wondered whether God would choose not to heal us.

The prospect of our disabilities being permanent was hard for our families to accept. Knowing it had been caused by the Pyridoxine overdose made it all the harder to bear. Equally troubling was the thought that the cost of our 24-hour care would be enormous. The Rehab staff and some of Denny's family began to talk to us about suing Dr. Palmer and Community Hospital. They said a terrible mistake had been made and somebody needed to pay for it. Without a large settlement, we would almost certainly end up in a nursing home with Russell being raised by someone else.

Neither Denny nor I wanted to sue, though. Life had become complicated enough already without the added stress of a lawsuit. We just wanted to forgive any wrongdoing and trust the Lord to provide for our future. We discussed our dilemma with many people. My family was not in favor of suing but recognized what we were up against and did not resist the idea. Pastor Lee and most of our church friends didn't seem to feel that suing would be scripturally wrong. One of them said, "Sometimes you have to do what you have to do." Only Darryl Edwards, who had joined Pastor Lee and Dad in anointing us on our first day in the hospital, said it would be wrong.

If our decision would have affected only Denny and me, we probably would have decided against a lawsuit. But there was little Russell to consider. Surely God wanted him to be with his parents. And our families would endure a great deal if they took responsibility for our care or if they saw us living in a nursing home separated from our son. In addition, we were reminded that doctors pay malpractice insurance for cases like ours. Would it be fair to everyone involved if we did not make use of that system of compensation?

Reluctantly, we agreed to let Kathryn contact a law firm and arrange a meeting. Soon afterward, she brought in two attorneys from a firm in a mid-Michigan city, Todd Baker and Luke Conway. We met them in the office of the head Rehab social worker, Martha Stavros. My parents, Kathryn, and Martha sat with us and the lawyers as we discussed the details of what had happened to us, the suspected cause of our neurological deficits, and the prognosis for our future. Todd and Luke felt our case warranted investigation, so we signed papers giving them the go-ahead. My signature was poor but legible; Denny signed with an X.

During the same meeting, we signed other papers giving power of attorney and guardianship of Russell to Kathryn. Although she had been handling our mail and finances and caring for Russell all along, she now had legal authority to do so. She had already needed to get medical attention for him once for multiple bee stings.

Denny and I left the meeting feeling beaten by our ordeal. We were both physically helpless, our child and all our affairs were in someone else's hands, and we felt forced to begin a lawsuit. We desperately wanted God to end it all through complete healing. With Dad and Pastor Lee's help, another anointing was arranged in the hospital chapel. Four pastors and my parents gathered around us for prayer and anointing.

But afterward, we saw no dramatic change in our conditions. Progress was being made, but it continued to be slow.

It was hard to accept that God was allowing our trial to go on. I knew he had not abandoned us, but I struggled to understand his reasons for all the pain. Denny, on the other hand, had reached his breaking point. He became angry with God, called him names, and told him he wanted to die. He tried to figure out how to get himself over to his tenth-story window and throw himself to the ground. But he could only lie on his bed watching the pigeons walk on the windowsill and feel resentful that God was allowing them to walk but not him.

Year: 2005

Dear Rehab staff,

Over the years I have come to appreciate the difficult job you do. The patients you work with have broken bodies, shattered dreams, and grieving hearts. They are confused and disoriented by all the loss and change. It must be hard to watch them go through that inevitable stage of denial before coming to terms with their new reality.

When you said we would need 24-hour care for life, it was devastating. Because the extent of our sensory deficits were unlike anything you had seen before, you had to make your prognosis based on what you knew about sensory loss in general. You were trying to brace us for the worst-case scenario even while we were all praying for the best.

I would like to make a suggestion that might help you in dealing with other patients whose physical deficits are unique. It would have been helpful in our case if you had presented us with this challenge: "Having no predecessor with this kind of handicap, you have the task of setting the standard for achievement for people with total sensory neuropathy. You show us what a person can do without touch. Not only that, we want to see what your God can do with someone who is willing to push the limits."

Thank you for being willing to do such a difficult job!

Sincerely,
Mae Jean Mason

Chapter 3

Adjustments

I only watch comedies," said my new roommate Jean as she flipped through the channels on our TV. "I need to laugh right now." A single mother of two young children, Jean had been left paralyzed from the waist down after having a tumor removed from her spinal column.

All of us in Rehab needed to laugh in order to cope with our problems. We made it a point to talk and joke about them as if they were no big deal. We went so far as to say we were all having a great time. Why, when it came right down to it, we were having more fun than human beings should be allowed. The staff encouraged us to laugh and to find whatever enjoyment we could in life. They joked with us often and helped us poke fun at ourselves. One time I overheard an occupational therapist playfully chiding two of her quadriplegic patients for not showing enough initiative in learning to use their remaining abilities.

"The two of you together don't have enough initiative to burp independently," she teased them.

Short trips away from the hospital also helped us enjoy life a little more. We were taken to the movies, to an art fair, and to a park for a picnic with our families. Once, we had a luau on the roof of the children's hospital next door. Nevertheless, we had to cope with reality.

One problem Denny and I faced was knowing what to do with our feelings for each other. For a long time we chose to maintain an every-man-for-himself approach simply because it was impossible to help each other. The staff was concerned by our apparent lack of interest in one another and thought our marriage was falling apart. But our attitude was only an emotional survival technique. And as our physical problems lessened, we began spending more time together.

The loneliness created by our temporary separation was greater for Denny than for me, which was not surprising since he was the one who had always needed more affection. Since I could not give it to him, our families and friends and even the nurses stepped in. The seven women who came on my birthday stood in a line to give him hugs. Gina also stopped by to visit him whenever she had a few minutes to spare. One day she stayed a long time, and Denny began to worry that he was keeping her from her work. When he told her it was okay to leave, she explained that she was not on duty but had come on her own time.

"I'm all yours, Denny," she said with a smile, casually resting her lovely face in her hands.

As he basked in the warmth of her friendship, Denny forgot he was married. If she had mentioned my name just then, he probably would have blinked and said, "Mae who?" But his love was still for me, and whenever we were together, he tried to find some physical way to show it. Sometimes he tried to hold my hand, but we couldn't feel each other's hand or maintain a good hold. If we took our eyes off our hands, they slid apart. It made the gesture meaningless to me, and I asked him not to do it anymore.

"Maybe if we could lie down on my bed together," he suggested. "I miss you so much, Mae Jean. If I could just be close to you . . ."

I thought we were still too pain sensitive and clumsy to make it work. But he really wanted to try, so I agreed to let the nurses (who thought it was a great idea) transfer me onto his bed. As I had feared, the pressure of being against each other was uncomfortable and we could hardly move. Denny didn't seem to mind, though. It was an emotional comfort for him just to have me by his side.

Love never used to hurt like this, I thought. Before, love had always been soft, tender, and spontaneous. Now being close was painful, awkward, and frustrating. After just a few minutes, I tearfully called for the nurses, and they took me back to my room. *It won't be like this forever,* I reassured myself. *Someday we'll be normal again.*

The person who spoke with me the most about the emotional side of our ordeal was Martha. A believer like us, she was caring and eager to help. Yet, she had to work with several patients at a time and carried the responsibilities of being the head social worker in Rehab. So she was often in a hurry, only able to give a limited amount of time to each patient.

Generally, Martha's comments and advice were very helpful. Sometimes, however, when she and I talked one-on-one, she would say things that confused and troubled me. She, like the rest of the staff, knew Denny was having a harder time coping than I was. As a result, they looked at me as the stronger one. Martha once quoted this Scripture verse to me, "Those to whom much is given much will be required.", and used it to place a larger share of responsibility on my shoulders to carry our family through the painful adjustment process. But she went beyond that one day when she was talking about our personalities.

"I like Mae Mason," she told me, "but I love Denny Mason!"

Without a doubt, he had a boyish charm and a great sense of humor even in the midst of his pain that captured the hearts of many staff members. Yet, I felt at times like he was being favored and less was expected of him than me. At the time, I said nothing but kept my feelings to myself.

In addition to emotional issues, the staff began talking to us about the practical issues we would face when we left the hospital. We needed to get used to being cared for by family members and/or hired attendants. We needed to learn how to live in a place that was not as wheelchair accessible as the hospital. We needed to think about transportation and how we would manage financially while we waited for a legal settlement.

To give us a taste of life in the real world, we were given a day pass away from the hospital with Denny's family. When Carl came to get us, he had to lift each of us from our wheelchairs and put us into the car, then put the chairs in the trunk. He took us to their house where Holly, their children, Kathryn, and Russell waited for us. We found that there were two steps at the front door to scale, the bathroom was not accessible, and there were no paved pathways around the yard (unlike the hospital). About two weeks later, we spent a weekend there. On this extended trip, we had to let Holly and Kathryn give us bed baths and clean up after bowel movements. Although they did these tasks cheerfully, it was more embarrassing having them done by family members than by hospital personnel.

We soon began making decisions about where and how we would live when released from Rehab. There was no way we could go back to our little second-floor house. Installing an elevator would be costly and take up precious space, and a ramp was not feasible. We had the option of living with my parents or Kathryn and chose to go to Mom and Dad's. The large parlor at the front of their old house could serve as a bedroom for Denny, Russell, and me. Also, the two of them could share the work of caring for us whereas Kathryn would have to carry the load alone. In addition, we decided to hire a personal care attendant to work eight hours per day to handle some of our care, and Dad began looking for someone to hire.

For transportation, we took all the money we had in the bank plus some donations from Denny's coworkers and bought a van. Carl shopped the dealerships in his area, picked out a van, and had a lift and wheelchair tie-downs installed. We considered the other types of expenses we would soon face and where we would get the money to cover them. Our hospital bills were being covered by Denny's health insurance; but once we left the hospital, we would have to pay for any further medical care, equipment, attendants' wages, and outpatient therapy in addition to ordinary living expenses.

Denny was receiving sick pay, and donations were coming in, the largest amounts coming from our congregation and Denny's coworkers. But we still needed a lot more. The two largest sources for obtaining government funds were Social Security and welfare. Martha and Kathryn helped us complete the paperwork for disability benefits first. An S.S. representative told us we would begin receiving checks six months from the onset of our disabilities, which meant October. We could not apply for welfare benefits until our own resources were depleted. Martha recommended taking Denny's name off the farm as soon as possible. If the farm were in Kathryn's name alone for more than a year before we applied for welfare, it would not have to be put up for sale. Martha believed our other personal resources, together with disability benefits and donations, would carry us through the first year.

Denny and I continued to make slow but steady progress both physically and emotionally. By early August, after having several roommates each, we wanted to try sharing a room again. So when Denny's last roommate left the hospital, I was moved in with him. We did much better this time and were able to encourage each other. By then, Denny's anger toward God was ebbing. He knew that only the Lord could deliver us from our ordeal. He couldn't shake his little fist in God's almighty face and at the same time expect God to answer his prayers. Together we tried to understand God's reasons for allowing us to suffer so much.

"Denny, I can't help thinking about Joni Eareckson and all that she went through. In her book she mentioned a Bible verse that helped her. It's the one about all things working together for the good of those who love God. Remember that one?"

"Yeah, I remember. I also remember what I went to the altar and prayed for the Sunday before we went into the hospital. I prayed that God would make me a better Christian." *That's right, he did,* I thought. There had to be a connection.

"Mae Jean, do you think he might be punishing me for past sins?" It surprised me to hear him say that.

"We have both asked for forgiveness of our sins and accepted Jesus. Why would God be punishing us?"

"I've done some pretty bad things in my life," he said dismally.

Denny had always had a tendency to feel guilty about everything. When he was in school and another student did something mischievous while the teacher was out of the room, Denny would feel that he should confess to it. I hoped this tendency was the reason for his unusual thinking.

Adjustments

In mid-August, we were given a weekend pass to Mom and Dad's. They had set up two old hospital beds in the parlor for us. They had hung colorful streamers and put a "Welcome" sign on the wall in a much-appreciated attempt to make our arrival feel like a real homecoming. But this was not our home; it was theirs. Our home was a little loft house on a berry farm, and we could never go back there to live again.

As the weeks passed, Denny became increasingly anxious to be with Russell full time. Moreover, he didn't feel his therapy was doing him much good anymore and felt the doctors were forcing him to stay in the hospital, which seemed more and more like a prison to him. Kelly, his primary nurse, asked me what I thought she could do to help him deal with his frustrations, but I wasn't able to give her many ideas. Finally, our doctors said he could go home.

"He really would benefit from more therapy," they told me. "But as long as he's fighting us we can't make much progress with him. Hopefully, he will continue to improve his strength and coordination with outpatient therapy."

Denny was discharged on August 28, exactly four months after entering the hospital. At that point, he was able to help dress himself, transfer into his wheelchair using a sliding board, and wheel himself around fairly well. Because he was still quite pain sensitive, he could not tolerate sitting on a hard toilet seat and therefore continued using a bedpan.

Soon after his release, I went to Mom and Dad's on another weekend pass. While I was there, we were asked to do an interview with the local newspaper. It felt strange to have the media's attention, but our unusual situation captured their interest. As first-time interviewees, we let the reporter direct the conversation. Her questions focused mainly on the nature of our disabilities and the prognosis for the future. Little attention was given to the suspected cause, and we did not tell her about the investigation of our treatment at

Community Hospital. We tried to be cheerful and used humor in discussing our problems. When the article was published, our financial needs were mentioned, and we soon began receiving donations from many caring people, most of whom we had never met.

Back at the hospital, my slow but steady progress continued. I had not regained the feeling in my mouth but was eating enough pureed foods to sustain me, so my feeding tube was finally removed. I also began to feed myself, though I was quite messy at it and needed to wear a bib. I could turn in bed from my side to my back and was almost strong enough to get into my wheelchair unassisted. In late September, the Rehab doctors said it was time to let me go. Although I was still benefiting from therapy, they felt it would be best for Denny, Russell, and me to be together and believed I would continue to improve with outpatient therapy. As I prepared to leave the hospital for good, Martha gave me some parting advice.

"I know your families and friends have really stood by you during this crisis," she said, "but you need to be aware that often the relationships a person has before becoming handicapped drift apart when the permanence of the handicap sinks in. Don't be surprised if some of your friends stop coming around. Some people just won't know how to relate to you as a handicapped person when they have always known you as a whole person."

"I can see how that could happen," I said thoughtfully. "But I don't think it will with our friends. They're such caring people."

"Well, just be aware of it. More importantly, you need to think about your relationship with Denny. I know it's hard because of your limitations, but the two of you need to find some way to express your love for each other." I knew she was right but couldn't imagine what we could do together with our numb, pain-sensitive, uncoordinated bodies.

Adjustments

"It's just that . . . without feeling, any kind of physical contact seems so empty. Even holding hands!"

"I know," she said sympathetically. "But promise me you'll look for some small ways—cards and flowers, anything—to show your love."

I promised but held a pessimistic view about whether we would succeed. Of one thing I was sure, though. We had vowed eight years before to stay together for better or for worse, in sickness and in health. Those vows were being heavily tested, but we were committed to keeping them no matter what. With the Lord's help, we would make it somehow.

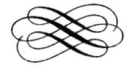

Life had not gotten easier for Denny during the four weeks between his discharge from the hospital and mine. Although he was glad to be with Russell again, he was still struggling to cope with his disability and the many problems it created. As a man, it was hard to accept being unable to work and support his family. He felt stripped of his strength and his position as head of his own household. He didn't like having to live under someone else's roof, and he became resentful of Dad, the able-bodied male in whose home he now lived.

In addition, tension was growing between our families, particularly our parents. It had begun when we had talked of moving Russell from Kathryn's home to Pati and Matt's. Then, the hardships everyone had endured throughout the long, hot summer had worn them down, making tempers grow short and the tension increase. Mom and Dad had driven to Ann Arbor countless times in addition to working and preparing to take us in. Kathryn had also made numerous trips to see us, cared for Russell, and managed the berry business with the help of a hired man. Through it all, they had watched in anguish as Denny and I suffered and had been heartbroken by the permanence of our disabilities. Everyone was under a great deal of emotional stress.

Whenever Ellen, our newly-hired care attendant, took Denny to visit his mother, he lamented about his life and how hard it was living with Mom and Dad. Kathryn began to think they were keeping him there against his will and wanted Denny and Russell to live with her instead. Additionally, the strong bond that had developed between Kathryn and Russell during their four months together made it hard for her to be separated from him. As a result, Denny and Russell began spending a few days at a time at her house. There, Denny didn't have a physically able male figure to feel resentful toward, and he found some comfort in being in his childhood home. But he still had to contend with his disability and shattered life. Those things could not be left behind.

In his depression, Denny stopped trying to make physical progress. He let Ellen or family members transfer him into and out of his wheelchair and do most of his dressing, even though he could do it himself when he left Rehab. He often lay in bed until 11:00 a.m. or later simply because he didn't feel there was anything to get up for.

Then the unexpected made matters worse. In Germany, trouble between my brother-in-law Dave and his Army superiors led to his sudden discharge. Sue, Dave, and their five children flew back to Michigan and, with no other place to go, moved in with Mom and Dad, too. There were two large empty bedrooms upstairs where they could stay. But now there were five adults, six children under eleven years of age, and an old half-blind dog all living in the same house. Sue and Dave started looking for work and a place to rent, but it took several weeks to find both. During that time, I was released from the hospital and joined a household of tense adults and

Adjustments

active kids. We were all caught in a tough situation that only time would change, and we had to make the best of it.

Our television, stereo, and our own beds had been moved from our house into the parlor/bedroom, and we spent a lot of time there listening to music and watching TV (mostly comedies, of course). We played Scrabble, and I put some puzzles together. These were old favorite pastimes and served as good hand therapy. Russell played with his cousins, went for walks in the woods with his grandpa, and went to Head Start. Denny and I were not able to do many things with him but enjoyed just having him near.

We read our Bibles and went to Sunday services as often as we could. Usually we went to my parents' church, but occasionally we visited our own congregation in Pleasant Creek 40 miles away. The first time we went back the congregation was so thrilled to see us that everyone stood and applauded our return. Then they whisked us to the front of the sanctuary to say a few words. It was painful going back as disabled people, and we didn't feel at all comfortable being the center of attention. So we kept our comments short and simple.

While living with Mom and Dad, we were asked to do another interview, this time with a much larger newspaper. The resulting article was eventually reprinted in at least four other newspapers around Michigan. Soon more donations started coming in, including an Amigo motorized cart that was given to us by the manufacturer.

After a while, Sue and Dave found jobs and a house and moved out, which eased some of the tension. Sadly, the interfamily conflicts continued, and hurtful things were sometimes said. Also, there was a debate over Ellen's ability as a care attendant. She did well on personal care but occasionally refused to do other tasks to help out around the house. Some family members pressured us to replace her, but we chose not to.

We were afraid it would be hard to find someone who would do as well on personal care.

It was hard to think about physical progress with so much to contend with emotionally. Nevertheless, I contacted the nearest hospital and made an appointment to begin outpatient therapy. It cost $45 per person per visit, and they wanted us to come in two or three times a week. It was more than we could afford, and after a few sessions we stopped going. A visiting nurse from the local Health Department who came to see us weekly knew about an in-home therapy program through the district Health Department whose cost was based on income. She checked into it for us, and soon we were getting affordable therapy at home.

Our income from disability and donations was more than enough to cover our present living arrangement. We saved our extra income toward eventually getting a place of our own with 24-hour hired care. Then in December we got a big boost from two fundraising events held by the community on our behalf. One was a small spaghetti dinner and the other was a huge auction/dinner/dance. Together they raised over $10,000. With such a large amount to draw upon, it was time to call the apartment complexes in Pleasant Creek to see if they had any handicapped units. One had three units, but they were all occupied. The manager had me fill out an application anyway to keep on file until there was a vacancy. We prayed that someone would move out soon.

During the months since leaving the hospital, our primary lawyer, Todd Baker, had visited us periodically and given us updates on his investigation. He told us there was no question that errors had been made in our treatment at Community Hospital. Not only had Dr. Palmer made judgment errors in Todd's opinion, but he also gave specific reasons for ascribing a degree of fault to the pharmacist, the hospital, the drug company, and the company that wrote the treatment instructions for the Poison Control Center. Dr. Palmer and his lawyers were contending that the nerve damage might have been caused by the mushroom poisoning, but the vitamin experts Todd had consulted were sure it was due to the Pyridoxine overdose.

It was all very complicated. Each party had contributed in some way—large or small—to our overtreatment. We knew we had a legitimate case but constantly debated whether or not it was morally acceptable to pursue a settlement. We just wanted to forgive everyone and put it all behind us. Yet, our needs were real and were not going away any time soon.

"It isn't right before God to sue," Denny told me. "How can we do this and still call ourselves Christians?"

"But the passage in 1 Corinthians about lawsuits is talking about suits between believers," I reminded him. "It doesn't say that all lawsuits are wrong."

"But we don't even know whether Dr. Palmer is a Christian brother or not!"

To my shame, I couldn't recall any meaningful conversations about spiritual matters with Dr. Palmer during the four years I had worked for him. I knew him to be a kind person, a fair boss, and a compassionate doctor, but was he a fellow believer? I didn't know.

"Besides," Denny went on, "even if he is an unbeliever, what kind of a witness is it to sue him?" It was a good question, but we had to consider our financial need. Our current resources would not last long, especially if we rented an apartment and hired 24-hour care. Without a settlement, we would eventually be forced into a nursing home.

"But God made the family unit," I argued. "I'm sure it's his will for us to stay together. Anyway, doctors pay malpractice insurance for cases like ours."

"Maybe God will heal us if we just have enough faith to trust him for the future. Then we wouldn't need any more money. And even if he didn't heal us and we went into a nursing home, at least we would have a clear conscience before God. Besides, I deserve to suffer for the terrible things I've done in my life," he added sorrowfully.

Denny wanted very much to drop the lawsuit, but I refused to agree. When we discussed our difference of opinion with Pastor Lee, he saw no problem, saying it was possible for God to lead one of us to go ahead and the other one to drop out. That didn't make sense to us. If it was wrong for one to sue, it was wrong for both. We then turned to Darryl Edwards for guidance. During the years that we had known him through the church, he had taught the Scriptures with authority and as one who knew the heart of God. We looked up to him as a Spirit-filled man.

Several times we called on Darryl for advice. He knew of other relevant Bible passages besides the one in 1 Corinthians. He shared them with us and explained their meaning. For Denny, they were confirmation of his beliefs, but I barely heard them. All I could think of was life in a nursing home, separated from Russell. Darryl was not unfeeling about our dilemma, and his compassion was evident. Once, as Denny and I passed the tissue box and dried our eyes, Darryl stared down at the open Bible in his lap.

"This is so hard," he said with a heavy sigh. But he continued to stand by the principles he saw in the Bible and discouraged us from suing.

"Remember that no matter what you decide to do God will still love you," he assured us.

Soon afterward Denny made a firm decision to drop the lawsuit, then called Todd at his law office and told him. Needless to say, Todd came to visit the very next day. I had resolved to press on no matter what Denny did, so during the visit I said little and just let Denny talk. He explained to Todd his conviction that it was morally wrong to sue.

"As a Christian myself, I think you are doing the right thing by suing," Todd countered.

Taken by surprise, Denny paused to think. Todd had much to gain financially by having us go forward, and in his mind Denny questioned Todd's beliefs and motives. We had met too many people for whom Christianity simply meant going to Sunday services and living a fairly clean life. Often they had little or no understanding of salvation and no personal relationship with the Lord.

"Under what definition do you call yourself a Christian?" Denny asked skeptically.

"I call myself a Christian because I have accepted Jesus Christ as my personal Savior," Todd answered with a knowing smile. His response gave more credibility to his claim and to his views.

He talked to us about the need for accountability among doctors and reminded us that the purpose of malpractice insurance is to compensate those who have been wrongfully injured. He felt it would be morally wrong to place the financial burden of our care on our families or the state welfare system. In addition, he said our case might turn out to be very important to those in the medical community who wanted to see greater governmental regulation of vitamins. It was possible for anyone to buy one-gram tablets of B-6 over the counter and potentially overdose himself at home. With Todd's persuasive arguments and without my support, Denny backed down. His change of heart was a relief but by no means a victory. I didn't want to sue either but felt we had no other choice.

As the winter progressed, we continued living with my parents with Denny and Russell spending short periods at Kathryn's. The visits by the occupational therapist and nurse ended because we no longer needed them, but we maintained our in-home twice-weekly physical therapy. To help fill time,

Denny bought a VCR and had it hooked to his mother's TV for watching rented movies. He also bought a Honda Odyssey for summer use. I didn't want him to spend so much on a nonessential, but he was desperate for ways to stay occupied, especially outdoors. To him, the Odyssey was a necessity.

Then in early February, an apartment opened up for us in Pleasant Creek, and we immediately began making arrangements to move in. We planned to hire three care attendants. A live-in attendant would care for us from 5:00 p.m. to 9:00 a.m., and two others would work days—one during the week and the other on weekends. We ran a "Help Wanted" ad and interviewed applicants. We also talked to church friends about moving our belongings—some from Mom and Dad's and some things still in our house at the farm.

During this busy time, we had an unexpected visitor from Children's Protective Services (CPS). Someone had told him Russell was not being cared for properly. He questioned us for a long time about our circumstances and left us with the impression that we had nothing to worry about. Still, it was a shock to think that someone considered us unfit parents. We knew CPS could take Russell away from us if they decided it was in his best interest. With both of us disabled, we felt like we had two strikes against us. A few days later Russell's Head Start teacher called. She had been questioned, too. She said she told the man, "Taking that little boy away from his parents is the worst thing that could happen to him!" Fortunately, we never heard from him again.

Moving day came on February 15. After our friends loaded our belongings at Mom and Dad's house onto their trucks, Denny went with them to the apartment while I went with other friends to the farm. I had been there only a few times since being discharged from Rehab, usually to have Ellen get something from inside the house. I couldn't help noticing how abandoned the farm looked, and it always made me feel

Adjustments

depressed to be there. On this trip, I went into the house for the first time. Two men carried me in my wheelchair up the stairs and into the dusty, unheated living quarters. They too looked abandoned. Most of our remaining possessions were in disarray from being sorted through whenever someone had searched for something we needed.

I gave my attention to the movers who needed to know which items to load and which to leave behind. In the process of giving instructions, I happened to glance up at the calendar on the wall. It was still turned to April. It was a stark reminder that the life we had known here had abruptly ended on that April morning when we left to go to the hospital. Almost ten months had passed since then. I hoped that in reestablishing a home of our own we would begin to feel like a family again and a degree of normalcy would return to our lives.

Year: 2005

Dear Martha,

Working with Rehab patients was different for you than for the medical staff members. They focused primarily on the physical while you focused on the practical and the emotional. In our case, your help was invaluable on the former but out of balance on the latter. Far more attention was given to staying strong and making life-strategy decisions than on grieving our losses and accepting our disabilities. Maybe you tried to talk to us about grieving and we didn't listen because we were still in a state of denial (as were those who made up our support system). Or maybe there just wasn't enough time.

More importantly, you were the first of many over the years to place more responsibility on me than on Denny for our family's survival. I should have told you how that made me feel. Back then, my personality often led me to quietly accept other people's expectations of me. But it was not beneficial to me nor to Denny. He needed to be encouraged to carry an equal share of the responsibility. I should have pressed him to make some of the calls for outpatient therapy and renting an apartment. It would have made him feel needed and would have taken some of the load off me.

Martha, I am still grateful today for your help and compassion. You did what you could before releasing us to the outside world. I want you to know that I have since learned to be more vocal about my own needs and feelings.

Thank you!
Mae Jean Mason

Chapter 4

Threshold

The first few weeks at the apartment were spent adjusting to managing our new home and getting acquainted with our new care attendants. I developed a work schedule and divided the housework, physical care, and errand running among them. All three attendants were certified nurse's aides in their early twenties. Our live-in attendant, Myrna, was an enthusiastic Christian and a sister-in-law to my younger sister Pam. Though overweight, she was energetic and constantly on the go. Our weekday attendant, Lynn, was married with two little girls. Sandy, who worked weekends, was married with no children and loved racy cars. We soon settled into a relaxed daily routine, and our emotional burdens eased somewhat. In addition, the tension between our families subsided as they saw us functioning well on our own and got their own households back to normal.

After about two months, we had to make a "staff" change. Lynn's baby sitter quit and she couldn't find a new one, so she left us to stay home with her girls. We moved Sandy to weekdays and hired Karen for weekends. As the weeks passed, we began to enjoy life a little more, and Denny joked ever more freely with Myrna, Sandy, and Karen. Although we still longed to be normal, we were thankful for the positive changes that were taking place. Our twice-weekly workouts with our therapist, Kay, became more productive, and we saw some physical improvements. Denny went back to dressing himself, doing his transfers, and wheeling himself around. He took the footrests off his chair so he could use his feet to help move himself around, too.

As our physical strength increased, Kay had us try walking with a walker. Denny was able to take several small steps as long as Kay held onto a strap tied securely around his waist and steadied the walker with her other hand. Denny was wobbly and walked like a drunk. He often played the part by slurring his words and saying things to Kay like, "Hi, honey. You married?" I was able to stand with the walker, but with my very limber knees, I did not have enough control to take a step.

Other physical changes were also taking place. Reduced pain sensitivity allowed Denny to tolerate sitting on the toilet, and he gladly bid farewell to the bedpan. Our increasing ability to compensate for touchlessness with our eyesight made simple tasks progressively easier. I became much neater when eating and tossed out the bib. We still had trouble sleeping because of our many aches and pains but were noticing that we felt less fatigued. And my reproductive system resumed its monthly cycles after nearly a year of inactivity.

But the spiritual turmoil created by the lawsuit did not let up. Occasional grumbling over modern medicine's overconfidence in itself and restatements of the legitimacy of our case didn't help. Denny wrestled over it constantly.

"How can I ever be happy," he once asked me, "with all that money and my family with me knowing that I neglected to do what was right in God's sight and then trust him to provide for the future?"

We had been over it many times, and I didn't know what more to say. He had continued to talk with Darryl about it until he had nothing more to offer either. I finally came to the conclusion that if it was tormenting him that much we might as well drop it. If he couldn't live with himself over it, it would be hard for Russell and me to live with him. More than staying together, I wanted him to be at peace with himself and with God. When I shared my conclusion with him, Denny was very relieved. Our conversations changed as we focused more attention on our mutual distaste for suing and on trusting the Lord—not the legal system—for help.

We wanted to break down the barrier erected by the legal investigation between ourselves and Dr. Palmer, so we gave him a call and invited him over. He came within a few days, bringing his wife and small son along. Laying aside the lingering questions about the overdose, Denny and I spoke primarily of our concern over the country's growing malpractice crisis, the outrageous settlements making headlines, and our desire to have no part in it. Our only reason for pursuing the lawsuit was our financial dilemma.

A few days later I called Todd. He soon came to see us and brought with him Luke Conway, his associate whom we had met in the hospital. We explained our position to them and then listened as they argued against it. The estimated cost for our 24-hour care, physical therapy, medical equipment, an accessible home and specialized van plus regular living expenses over the next 30-40 years was $2 million. Medical experts they had consulted agreed with their estimate. Disability benefits, welfare, and donations would not be enough. Family men themselves, Todd and Luke showed genuine concern for our family and wanted to see us stay together. They did not pressure us to seek more than economic damages, though Todd believed a jury would probably award us $20 million for pain and suffering.

I listened quietly to all they had to say, but inside I was yelling, "I don't want to sue! I don't want to live in a nursing home! I don't know what to do!" In the end, it was Denny's decision since he was struggling the most over it. When the discussion ended, he reluctantly told them to carry on with the case.

Before leaving, Todd asked us not to contact Dr. Palmer again. For the other side to know we wanted out was going to make his job harder. The other side's lawyers were acknowledging by then that errors had been made but now would probably drag their feet in making out-of-court settlements on the chance we might yet drop the suit. Though we understood Todd's reasoning, his request was an unwelcome restraint. I called Dr. Palmer one more time anyway to let him know we were going ahead for financial reasons, and he said he understood. Afterward, Denny and I agreed that we needed to learn to live with the lawsuit—like it or not—and stop debating it.

Spring came and with it an intense longing to pick up where we had left off the year before, living at the farm and working in the fields. I felt a deep sadness come over me as I watched nature renew itself and wished that we could be renewed, too.

We noticed Russell becoming more open about his own struggle to cope with our disabilities. "Why did you guys eat those mushrooms anyway?" he often asked angrily. Sometimes his frustration over small things would bring his deep feelings to the surface, and he would physically strike out, almost always at Denny. We hurt for him as well as for ourselves when we thought of all the things we could no longer do with him—camping, biking, swimming. Nor could we give him little brothers and sisters. And it was difficult to watch someone else bandage his wounds when he got hurt instead of caring for him ourselves.

When summer came, we spent time out in the sunshine and started concentrating more on what we *could* do. Denny took an interest in the little children at the apartment complex who played with Russell. Most were from single-parent households and didn't see their fathers much, causing them to respond warmly to Denny's friendship. He liked to organize them into a cleanup crew, pick up the scrap papers around the complex, and then treat them to candy bars or popcicles. A few times an attendant helped him take Russell and some of the older boys fishing. Occasionally Denny and Russell were taken to the farm to ride around in the Odyssey.

Since we were now attending our home church's services regularly, we wanted to find a way to become actively involved again. When we learned that a position called Moral Issues Director was open, we asked for and received permission to try it. Our job was to research the prominent moral issues of the day and report periodically to the congregation about them. I went to a Christian book store, picked out several books on current issues, and started reading.

Around this time, the unexpected happened again. One evening a while after supper, Denny mentioned that he was feeling sick to his stomach. Myrna and I were nauseous, too. Denny and Myrna agreed that the meat for supper had tasted strange. Because my meat and vegetables had been pureed together, I had not noticed the funny taste. Fortunately, Russell had not eaten any meat. All night long Myrna cared for Denny who stayed in bed utilizing a basin and a bedpan. Though I remained very nauseous all night, I held my supper down. Poor Myrna might have fared the same if she had not been cleaning up after Denny. In the wee hours of the morning, she came to me to talk about Denny's condition.

"I'm getting worried about him," she said. "He's not getting any better. I told him I thought he should go to the hospital, but he says he's not going back there." I understood his feelings all too well.

"I'm sure not going to tell him to go," I replied. "Whatever he decides is fine. If he wants to wait it out here, that's up to him."

As day dawned, Denny had Myrna call Darryl and ask him to come over to pray with him, which Darryl gladly did. Soon his vomiting and diarrhea stopped. We thanked God that Denny had not repeated the three days of vomiting we had experienced with the mushroom poisoning.

With this minor crisis behind us, I resumed my reading. The first book I had chosen was about abortion. I had always been against it but had never looked into the issue before. I was appalled by what I learned through the book, and it struck me full force that abortion kills a little person. The methods used to kill unborn children would be considered inhumane for executing convicted criminals or even destroying unwanted animals.

After finishing the book, I had a heavy burden for the unborn, for their mothers who are often uninformed, and for society because of its apathy over the self-inflicted loss of its children. I wrote an essay about abortion and distributed it within our church. The response was limited but encouraging, and I started learning about antiabortion legislation in order to keep the congregation up-to-date. Although Denny didn't read the book, he showed a strong interest in the issue and worked closely with me. He clearly had a burden for the unborn, too, and sometimes became tearful when talking about abortion.

As the summer wore on, our financial reserves dwindled, and we began selling possessions. We sold the Chevette, the Ford pickup with its snow plow, the front-end loader Denny had bought for farm use, his hunting rifles and his scuba gear. We were no longer using these things, but it was hard to let them go since each one represented an important part of our former lifestyle.

It took a lot of effort at times not to be depressed. Sometimes the weight of our physical and emotional battle felt like it would crush us, and we pleaded with God to heal us. We had some encouragement to do so from our loved ones. Many times we were told, "If only this hadn't happened to you." They, too, were struggling to accept the permanence of our handicaps. The most influential voice was Darryl's. He said that according to the Bible, a believer's request for healing should always be answered with a "yes" and believed that something was holding up our prayers in the spiritual realms. As a result, we asked Pastor Lee to anoint us yet again. The next Sunday many people stayed after services to join in a special prayer time for us. But a miraculous healing didn't happen, and we went home to face the same struggles.

One day, Denny brought up his past sins again.

"You know, Mae Jean, I've done some pretty bad things in my life," he said sadly. Why did he keep saying that? Why not forget the past instead of allowing it to make the present even more burdensome? Then he let me know for the first time that he was referring to a specific incident.

"Mae, I did something a long time ago—before we met—that I've never told you about." He paused for a moment. "I really want to tell you about it, but I'm afraid that if I do you'll leave me."

I had no idea what he was talking about and wasn't sure I wanted to find out. Whatever it was, it had to be pretty bad if he thought it had the potential to break up our marriage.

"Do you think I should tell you?" he asked uncertainly.

"I . . . don't know, Denny."

He chose to say no more, but my imagination went into high gear as I tried to figure out what he might have been keeping from me all those years. I could only speculate and did so endlessly. I asked no questions but waited for him to tell me about it when he was ready.

With Kay's help on our physical therapy, we were gaining strength, stamina, and coordination and were able to get out of the apartment regularly. Consequently, Kay told us we no longer qualified for in-home therapy and stopped coming. Knowing the high cost of outpatient therapy, we chose to maintain an exercise routine at home with only the help of our attendants.

Subtle problems were developing in our live-in arrangement with Myrna. Our apartment was small, and the belongings of a fourth person made it more crowded. Additionally, the extra visitors and phone calls that went with her active lifestyle were sometimes disruptive. Denny and I decided to eliminate the live-in position and instead have attendants working three eight-hour shifts. We changed the schedule in early August putting Sandy on the 7:00 a.m. to 3:00 p.m. shift and Myrna the 3:00 to 11:00 p.m. shift five days each. Karen got the four leftover mornings and evenings. Since the 11:00 p.m. to 7:00 a.m. shift involved little work, we hired my sister Pam, who was attending college by day, to work five nights a week. The other two nights went to Rhonda. Both new workers were married with a small daughter.

Around this time, we experienced another minor crisis. Russell, now four and a half, had learned to ride another child's bike without training wheels, and we proudly bought him a shiny, new two-wheeled bike. We enjoyed watching him ride but noticed that he, like the other children, often failed to stop at the end of the cement handicap ramp before riding into the parking lot. An elderly man parked his truck next to it, making it impossible for a child to see any oncoming cars until reaching the end of the ramp. One day when Karen and I were in the living room, she glanced out the window and suddenly stiffened.

"Oh, my God! Someone just hit a child!" she cried, bolting out the door.

Because the handicap ramp was almost directly in front of our living room, I knew right away what had happened. A moment later she returned carried a sobbing Russell. He had ridden his bike into the front quarter panel of an oncoming car. A half second sooner and he would have ridden into its path. On impact, he was knocked off his bike and scraped his back on the cement. He had no other injuries. We thanked God once again for his intervention.

Although Karen was good with Russell that day, she was often borderline abusive with him. Denny talked to her about it a couple of times to no avail, and after a while we chose to let her go. It was a hard decision because she was good on physical care and needed the job, but we didn't need the extra stress that her negative attitude toward our son created. Our other attendants worked her shifts until we hired Lois to replace her. Single and about 20, Lois became the latest addition to our personal staff.

During August, a company that had been questioned but cleared in Todd's investigation gave us $5,000 to help out. Then several weeks later one of the parties implicated in the investigation agreed to an out-of-court settlement. At that point, we had enough cash in the bank to last about a month. We had been able to hold on to several of our possessions, including the four acres, and had not applied for welfare.

The settlement seemed large but was only a fraction of our projected need. Our lawyers deducted their expenses and fees, and a small portion was set aside for Russell's college education. The rest of the money was put into an annuity and would be paid back to us in a fixed monthly amount.

Combined with our disability benefits, it would cover our monthly expenses for the next four years. By then, Todd was confident that other settlements would be reached, our financial future would be secure, and all would be well—that is, financially. The settlement brought us only limited peace. There was still the lingering feeling that we were not choosing the right path. Although the money was going to keep us together, it couldn't make us happy.

Without touch, I was having a hard time relating to other people in any meaningful physical way. I could not feel handshakes, and hugs were not comforting. When someone hugged me, I could not sense the softness of his/her body or even my own. I could only sense pressure against my bones, making me feel like nothing more than a skeleton. And my poor coordination made it hard to hug someone back. For Denny, the need for affection overshadowed these problems. He found some comfort in just seeing that he was being hugged. In trying to be close to each other, the differences in our emotional responses to touchlessness caused tremendous frustration.

I wondered what the future really held for us. Could Denny and I live together contentedly without giving or receiving any physical expressions of love? Time alone would tell. I put my hope in the Lord, believing he would work everything out for the good in his time.

One night I had an unusual dream. It came during the time when several Americans were being held hostage in Lebanon. In the dream, I was also a hostage being held in a small, austere room. The door opened, and a man in military clothing entered the room and approached me. Two guards stood outside the door.

"I have been given authority to give you any one thing you want except your freedom," he said. I thought carefully about what I wanted most. Then, as tears filled my eyes, I gave him my answer.

"All I really want is a hug."

He hesitated only briefly, then stepped forward and wrapped his muscular arms gently around me. It was only a dream, but I could actually feel his arms and the softness of his flesh. I had missed this simple comfort so much. I laid my head on his shoulder and softly cried.

As I later pondered the meaning of this brief but powerful dream, I realized that I viewed God as my captor, holding me hostage in the confines of my disabled body. But he had shown me through the dream that although he would not give me my freedom, I could turn to him for what I needed most—comfort.

Because our disabilities prevented us from working or being physically active, we had a lot of free time on our hands. Our involvement at church filled some time but not enough, and we looked for more things to do. In September, each of us enrolled in a night class through the high school. He took English, and I took Conversational Spanish. He also started taking Russell and his little friends across the street to the elementary school for an area church's program for children. Since writing by hand was difficult for me, I rarely wrote letters until a former coworker gave me her old typewriter. I couldn't type very fast without feeling the keys and had to watch my hands closely to be sure I was hitting the right ones, but it was faster and easier than handwriting. It felt good to keep in touch with friends at a distance again.

Also in September, Myrna decided it was time to move on and gave us two weeks' notice. Soon we hired Linda to replace her. A chubby girl of 19, she admitted during the interview that she was mentally slow. But she had completed a nurse's aide course and received her certification, so we gave her a chance. It took more time to train her than the others, but once trained she did fine. Later in the fall, Sandy also gave us two weeks' notice. Marital problems had caused her to leave home and then to a decision to leave the area. With five employees, Denny and I learned to expect to make staff changes regularly.

After receiving the settlement, we no longer qualified to live in the federally-subsidized, low-income apartment complex. Fortunately, the manager did not pressure us to move out quickly. Nevertheless, we began right away to look for a house to rent, preferably in the country. In December, we found a roomy house on Morley Road just two and a half miles from the farm. The owner allowed us to make small accessibility modifications in the house and build a ramp at the side door in the garage. On the 19th, Lois and her boyfriend moved our small possessions from the apartment, and two friends from the factory moved the big ones. We also had the appliances and some other belongings moved in from our old house. With a fresh helper every eight hours, unpacking went fast, and we were soon settled into another home.

After Sandy left, Myrna filled in part-time for several weeks followed by a new girl for about a month. Eventually, we hired Gina, a young married woman with a baby girl who loved riding horses, as Sandy's permanent replacement. Our revised staff—Gina, Linda, Lois, Rhonda, and Pam—was fairly stable, and we didn't need to make another change for several months.

With our night classes over, Denny and I had more free time again. We spent a lot of time reading our Bibles and sharing with our attendants. Because we talked openly with them about our struggles, they opened up to us about theirs, too. We shared our faith with them and encouraged each one to grow in her faith. Other than the attendants, we didn't have many people to talk to. Relatives visited occasionally, but visits from friends in the church or the factory were uncommon. We knew we could call on them if we needed something, but otherwise we rarely saw them.

It was sad to see that our factory friendships were fading, but I was dismayed that our church friendships were as well. Had Martha been right? Were our friends, even our Christian friends, having a hard time relating to us as handicapped people? We could do so few things with them now, but we still needed them. Perhaps they didn't understand that. Maybe we tried too hard to be cheerful on Sunday mornings and didn't let on to just how much we needed for them to spend time with us.

Our primary involvement with our congregation was still the Moral Issues directorship, and we continued to focus mainly on abortion. In the spring, when Right to Life of Michigan (R.L.M.) organized an initiative petition drive to end tax funding of abortion, we helped distribute petitions and related information to most of the churches in our county. It was our first countywide project, and it was an exciting experience. We were thrilled when our final signature count was well over R.L.M.'s goal for our area.

As the months passed, our physical strength and ability slowly improved as a result of our self-prescribed exercises and activities. Denny found that he could get down on the floor and back into his chair unassisted. He then started working out more vigorously on a mat on his bedroom floor. He also bought a three-wheeled bicycle. He had his brother John put a boat seat on it with a seat belt, and he had someone else put straps on the pedals so his feet couldn't slip off. It was incredible to watch him, his body strapped to the bike, going for rides with Russell. Though I lagged behind in progress, I was also making gains. There were a lot of linoleum floors in the rented house, which made wheeling around easier for me, and I began to do most of my own wheeling. I was also dressing myself and transferring into and out of bed without assistance.

Denny's ability to get down on the floor opened up new play opportunities for him and Russell. Of utmost fun was playing with Russell's Hot Wheels cars. They raced their cars around in a little circle within Denny's reach and often crashed them into one another intentionally. Then they had to take their cars to the pretend repair shop.

"Fix, fix, fix," Denny mumbled as he worked on his car. "Hammer, hammer, hammer. Repair, repair." Russell followed suit, mumbling and giggling as they worked.

"I's ready! You ready?" Denny hollered after a moment or two.

"Ready, Dad!" Russell beamed back, and they went at it again.

Although it was still difficult being parents in wheelchairs, we were learning to appreciate the simplest moments shared with our son. Watching him grow, sharing his excitement over losing his first tooth, and reading stories to him were special moments. Equally special were his antics. One incident happened when he stayed overnight with Kathryn. They went to the farm, and while they were there Russell found a bird's nest. When Kathryn brought him home, she waited until he was out of earshot before telling me about it.

"There were some eggs in the nest and he wanted to take one, but I wouldn't let him. He wasn't too happy with Grandma, but I didn't want him to disturb the nest. By the way, I wanted to let you know he had a little accident; he wet himself. He doesn't normally do that, does he?"

At five and a half, he had gotten past accidents long ago. Later in the day, however, after she had left, I heard the rest of the story. I was sitting at the dining room table when Russell came up to me and started talking about the nest he had seen at the farm.

"Grandma told me I couldn't take any of the eggs," he said, and then with a twinkle in his eyes he added, "but I took one anyway."

"You did?" I said casually, trying to cover my surprise at his confession. "What did you do with it?"

"I put it in my pocket. But on the way back to Grandma's house, it hatched! I got wet stuff on my pants. So when we got to Grandma's house, I told her I peed my pants, and she put them in the dryer."

I was having a hard time containing my laughter. Gina, working close by, was obviously having the same problem. Then he concluded his little story with a look of mischievous delight.

"I'll bet that birdie is flying around in Grandma's dryer right now!"

Gina and I lost our composure, and we laughed until we cried. What a privilege to live in the same house with this special little boy.

As Pam's July graduation from nursing school approached, Denny and I talked about what we would do afterward since she intended to leave us to get a nursing job. We found ourselves considering what had once been unthinkable: not hire a replacement and eliminate the night shift. The big question was whether we could handle being alone at night. Denny had a phone next to his bed with one-button dialing for emergency numbers, and we were both able to get into our wheelchairs and out of the house via the ramp.

We boldly decided to try it. We created a new schedule with two seven-hour shifts—one from 7:00 a.m. to 2:00 p.m. and the other from 3:00 to 10:00 p.m. We would be alone for nine hours at night and an hour between shifts in the afternoon. Because of the change, Rhonda's hours were being cut to just 14 per week, and she decided to get a different job. She left in June, and Pam left in July. Lois, Linda, and Gina remained to work the new schedule.

It felt strange not having an attendant in the house at night but not at all frightening. It was very natural, and we were thrilled over regaining such a large measure of independence. Financially, the change constituted a thirty percent cut in our wage expense, which meant the money from the settlement was going to last possibly as much as a year longer than originally anticipated. More importantly, the achievement was evidence that our Rehab doctors had been wrong. We did not need 24-hour care for life. Suddenly, the door to the impossible was open, and we were crossing the threshold. Only God knew for sure how far we could go.

Year: 2005

Dear Lord,

Thank you so much for allowing us to reach such a monumental goal. You made it possible for us to achieve more within the framework of our handicaps than we thought we could. I wish we would have stopped praying for complete healing at that point and focused all our energy on reaching our greatest physical potential just as we were. But you know how influential other people can be, especially those we love and respect, especially someone like Darryl who was such a wise and discerning believer. We trusted his judgment more than anyone else's. It was appropriate for him to be honest with us about his personal beliefs regarding healing. The problem was that we had so little confidence in *our* ability to discern your will in that area.

The message of the dream seems quite clear in hindsight. I believe you were trying to tell me that you were not going to give us the complete healing we sought. We didn't listen to the message, accept our "confinement", and embrace your comfort to the fullest extent possible. But in all honesty, I don't recall telling anyone about the dream back then. Would they have interpreted it as I now have even if they had known about it? I am so sorry, Father, for not listening to your still small voice or revealing the dream to others. If I had, we might have stopped wrestling over the healing issue and saved ourselves a lot of unnecessary distress later on.

Your grateful servant,
Mae Jean

Chapter 5

Revelations

In spite of our life-changing physical achievement, the lawsuit continued to cast a shadow over our lives. No other settlements had been reached, and Todd had filed the suit at the county courthouse. Soon depositions would be taken and a trial date set. We tried not to talk about it too much or agonize over it. Then one day Lois came to work with a bit of unwelcome news.

"Have you seen this week's paper?" she asked.

"No. Why?" I asked curiously.

"You guys made the front page."

Lois brought the newspaper to me and pointed to a small article entitled "Masons Suing Palmer, Community Hospital". We had told Todd we wanted the lawsuit kept quiet so as not to hurt the reputations of the doctor and hospital. But someone at the *County Blab* had gotten hold of the information. Now, there it was in black and white for all to read. The article gave few details, but the damage was done.

Surprisingly, the article brought out greater feelings of concern for ourselves than for anyone else. It was our own reputation as believers that was being hurt by the publicity, and it made us sick at heart. The lawsuit went against everything the Bible taught us—turn the other cheek; forgive and you will be forgiven; repay no one wrong for wrong; bless those who hurt you. The lawsuit had just ripped a gaping hole in the fabric of our Christianity. Denny had been right. How could we do this and still call ourselves Christians? Our discussions about it became filled with expressions of disgust. We wanted to encase the whole loathsome mess in cement and throw it into the nearest river.

Denny firmly told me he was going to draw the line at the courthouse door. If no other settlements were reached before the trial began, he would refuse to go through with it. He made his intentions known to Todd on his next visit, but Todd was not concerned.

"Denny, I'll talk you through this thing one step at a time," he said with a confident smile. Denny did not reply, but the look on his face spoke for him.

Around the same time, Denny again brought up his past. Instead of hinting at it as before, he chose to give me a clue.

"You know, Mae Jean, before we got married, I know you wanted to marry someone who had saved himself like you did. Well, I didn't. I wasn't a virgin when we got married. But it was just one time," he added quickly. "I knew it was wrong, but I did it anyway, and I hated it." I waited a moment in case he wanted to say something more.

"Okay, Denny. I can handle that," I said.

Was that it? Was this the dark sin he thought would break up our marriage? Certainly, it was important because it meant he had lied to me, but it wasn't worth throwing away ten good years of marriage over. I felt there had to be more but didn't ask. Not long afterward, his past came up again from an odd angle. We were sitting at the table talking, and the subject of capital punishment came up. I said I believed it was appropriate in cases of premeditated murder with irrefutable proof.

"Not me," he said, shaking his head, "because that would include me."

"What?! What are you talking about?"

"I had a hand in a murder once. I'd bring condemnation down on myself if I agreed to that." I stared at him for a moment, then shook my head.

"I don't believe that," I laughed. Realizing how strange his comments had sounded, he tried to clarify them.

"Well, it wasn't like . . ." and he gestured as though stabbing someone with a knife. "Nothing like that." I watched him closely to see if he was going to say more. He looked around the room. Both Lois and Russell were nearby.

"Let's go down to your bedroom to talk," he said.

I made my way down the hall to my room and transferred onto my bed to rest while he talked. I sensed that he was actually about to tell me what had been burdening him for so long. At the table, Denny took a deep breath. He was not going to put it off any longer, no matter what the consequences. He wheeled himself into my room and closed the door. Putting one foot up on the edge of the bed and crossing his forearms over his knee, he began to speak.

※

During his youth, Denny had felt pressured by his peers, the media, and his own desires to find out what sex was all about. He knew it was wrong outside of marriage and resisted for years, but he eventually gave in to it. He was 22 years old when he had an encounter with a young woman named Anna, the sister of two of his friends. Recently separated from her husband, Anna and her children were spending most of their time with her parents and brothers who lived near Denny's family home. His sexual relationship with her was not based on love but on his desires and her loneliness. She was a nice person and Denny got along well with her little ones, but their relationship brought him no happiness, only guilt and self-condemnation.

Then Anna became pregnant. They were caught off guard and didn't know what to do. He felt he should offer to marry her, but his parents didn't like her or her family. Without their support, he didn't think a marriage would work and ruled out that option without ever telling them about the pregnancy. It was 1975, and abortion was a legally permissible option. Feeling they had no other choice, Denny and Anna agreed to pay half each, and her brother Jake said he would drive her to the abortion clinic. Denny only saw her once after that.

The guilt he felt over his sexual immorality was made ten times worse by having contributed to the death of his own child. He became very depressed, and his feelings of self-worth plummeted. A year went by before he fell to his knees under the birch trees at the back of the farm and begged God to send him a wife, someone with whom he could have a right relationship.

I was surprised by how relaxed Denny was as he shared this dark chapter from his past with me. He apparently wanted to get it out in the open and was prepared to handle any kind of reaction. I was also surprised by my own calmness on learning about Anna and realizing that he had lied many times over the years in order to keep their relationship hidden from me. I understood now why he had felt his past would threaten our marriage. If I had learned of it before the overdose, I would have been deeply hurt and angry that he had not been honest about something so important. But our relationship had since changed. We no longer shared physical intimacy, so we had come to think of each other as companions first and lovers second. It was my friend more than my husband who sat near me in his wheelchair unloading his burden.

    I did not become angry or upset with him over his past. Instead, I felt sorry that he had carried the burden alone for so long, knowing I would not have been able to handle hearing it. We had been through a lot together in the last two years. The distant past was not important; finding peace for the present was. For Denny, peace would come in knowing that I loved him in spite of his past and forgave him for keeping it from me. Although he already knew the Lord had forgiven him, he needed to feel my forgiveness, too. I assured him that everything was okay; he didn't need to let it weigh him down any longer.

    In the following days, it was wonderful to see how happy and peaceful Denny was. I promised myself never to let resentful feelings about his past creep in and destroy my forgiveness of him. When we ask the Lord for forgiveness, he no longer holds our sins against us and does not hold us accountable for them (although the consequences of our choices often remain). Being able to forgive Denny in that way made me feel warm inside.

    But the lawsuit! I thought suddenly. *We've been saying that we forgive Dr. Palmer and the others, but our actions aren't demonstrating it. We're still holding them accountable by expecting them to pay financially for their mistakes.*

    Based on our memories from Community Hospital and the information obtained in the investigation, Denny and I had come to believe that the overdose had resulted mainly from overconfidence in vitamin therapy and judgment errors on the side of "trying too hard". While this did not excuse anyone's bad choices, it made feelings of forgiveness become stronger. Suddenly I saw how important it was to demonstrate our forgiveness by dropping the lawsuit.

It was quite exciting to think of it. There would be peace and freedom in total forgiveness. As for the future, I felt ready to trust God for that. He had been teaching us through our sufferings, and now a big lesson about forgiveness had been learned through the revelation of Denny's past. If we let the suit go and God chose to allow our family to suffer more, it would be for a reason. When I shared my thoughts and conclusion with Denny, he agreed wholeheartedly but hesitated to believe that we could actually drop it.

"If we call Todd, he'll just come here and talk us out of it again," he said pessimistically.

"I've thought about that, Denny, and I think there is a way to prevent it from happening. If we show Todd that our decision is final, he won't bother coming here to try to change our minds. And I really don't want to see him waste any more of his time on our case than he already has. I think if we send Todd a letter instead of calling him and tell him that we're dropping the lawsuit and why and then send copies of the letter to Dr. Palmer and the hospital—"

"Oooh," Denny breathed and gave me a sidelong look. "That would do it. But isn't that playing dirty?"

"I know it might seem that way at first, but I really think it's the best way. If I put a notation at the end of the letter that copies are being sent to Dr. Palmer and Community Hospital, Todd will know it's over. There won't be any point in coming here again." Denny thought for a moment.

"Okay," he said with a confirming nod. "Will you compose the letter?" I nodded in response. Then he extended his right hand toward me.

"Put 'er there, partner," he grinned, and we shook on it. We knew the days ahead would be filled with challenges, beginning with the inevitable criticism we would receive for making this decision. But we believed we were on the right track and sensed that blessings would follow.

Soon I began composing the most difficult letter I had ever written—a carefully worded letter to a lawyer who had spent countless hours on a case he felt was morally right. Although Todd had known all along how uncomfortable we were with the suit, I knew our letter would upset him. I tried to explain the reasons for our decision and thanked him for all his hard work on our behalf. We offered to pay for any expenses he had incurred since the settlement and told him why we were sending copies of the letter to the doctor and hospital. When it was finished, Lois made the copies for us in town, and we put them in the mail.

I was nervous in anticipation of Todd's reaction as I watched the mailman take the envelopes from the mailbox. My nervousness increased the next day as I envisioned Todd's secretary opening the letter, handing it to him to read, and then Todd angrily reaching for the phone. Sure enough, in the late morning the phone rang, and it was Todd. He said sending those copies was totally wrong; he felt betrayed; we should have given him a chance to talk to us first. And did we realize what this meant—going on welfare and living in poverty for the rest of our lives? I made little attempt to defend our decision. He was too upset at the moment to objectively consider our reasons.

To our surprise, he wanted to visit us. He felt he deserved an opportunity to express his viewpoint. When he came, he went over the familiar pro-lawsuit arguments, but we felt no pressure to change our minds. Maybe it was due to the strength of our resolve or the damage done by the copies or both. We were sorry that he had invested so much time in our case. Even though we had offered in the letter to pay for any new expenses, Denny went further and offered to give him any money we still had left from the settlement. I could tell from Todd's expression, however, that the offer was not well received.

"Don't take what I have been able to get for you and throw it back in my face," he said. He had been trying earnestly to help us, not just make money for himself through legal fees. Denny's well-intentioned offer was taken as an insult.

We told Todd about the newspaper article, its effect on us, and the spiritual lesson learned through the revelation of Denny's past. The nervousness we felt due to his displeasure with us caused us to talk a mile a minute, and it didn't seem to me that we were making things any clearer for him. By the end of our conversation, though, it was apparent that he had gotten something out of our nervous chatter. As he stood to leave, he looked momentarily out the window and then back at us.

"I guess you two have had more to deal with than I realized," he said.

Soon afterward we told our families what we had done. Denny was not ready to tell them about his past, so we simply told them we had dropped the lawsuit and were trusting God for the future. And so, although they had also known all along of our discomfort over the suit, they had no idea why we had suddenly let it go after more than two years.

Kathryn was the most upset and talked of going to Todd herself to resume the case on Russell's behalf. We did not want her to but knew we would answer to God only for our own choice, not for anyone else's. Dad was surprised by our decision and impressed by the strength of our faith. Mom remained silent, but we knew from previous discussions how concerned she was for our future. When Pati and Matt got the news, they came to see us and brought a box of home-canned foods as a symbol of their support.

Two people from Denny's family and Todd assumed that our church had convinced us to do it. We assured them that this was not the case. On the contrary, those individuals from our congregation with whom we had discussed the lawsuit had not opposed it. The only exception was Darryl, and we had not talked to him about it in months. The decision was ours alone.

Having done what we felt was right, we experienced a great peace. If God allowed hard times to come as a result of our decision, we knew he would have a purpose in them and teach us through them. We also felt a resurgence of an inner strength that came from knowing our circumstances did not have control over us but with God's help we were going to triumph over them.

We began to look at our situation from a different perspective. With no help coming in the future from additional settlements, we asked the Lord to show us how to make the most of the financial, physical, and mental resources we already possessed. We looked at our living expenses to see where we might make cuts and made an appointment with Michigan Rehabilitation Services (M.R.S.) to talk about possible vocational retraining.

On the day I was scheduled to see the M.R.S. representative, we had a final meeting with Todd. He and a lawyer from Grand Rapids who had been advising him on our case were planning to go to the courthouse to withdraw the lawsuit. The other lawyer wanted to meet us first. We had heard about him from Todd many times and knew he was considered one of the best lawyers in the state. We assumed he would make a final appeal to reverse our decision. We could only imagine his powers of persuasion, but we felt strong in spirit and determined to stand firm.

A distinguished man, the Grand Rapids lawyer greeted us warmly and complimented me on the composition of our letter. Then came the tough arguments. Appealing first to our Christian concern for others, he said that if we didn't feel comfortable taking lawsuit money for ourselves, we could use it to help the poor. But we said "no". If we would allow them to talk to the other side one more time, he was certain they would be more than happy to settle for $100,000. Again we said "no". Other arguments were presented, and still we held our ground. Finally, he appealed to our feelings as parents.

"What will Russell say someday," he asked Denny, "after growing up in poverty and he finds out what you have turned down?" It was a powerful question, but Denny was confident as he gave his answer.

"Russell will say that his parents lived by their convictions."

Soon the lawyers left, and we breathed a sigh of relief. After their visit to the courthouse, the lawsuit was finally over.

When I met with the M.R.S. representative later in the day, she and I discussed the nature of our disabilities and reviewed our educational backgrounds. When Denny saw her two weeks later, she recommended moving to a handicapped-living complex in Ann Arbor where we could be a little more independent at home and take classes at the university. We didn't want to move to a city, though, nor be so far from our families. We decided to hold off on retraining until we had reduced our monthly expenses as much as possible.

The biggest hindrance to further wage cuts was my need for help in the bathroom. Denny had become independent in that area by putting grab bars by the toilet. Because of my limber joints, I didn't have enough stability to stand up holding the bar with one hand while repositioning my slacks with the other. So we began to brainstorm for a solution.

During the weeks following our big decision, we made two staff changes. Linda moved out of the area, and Gina quit when she became pregnant with her second baby. Their replacements were Brenda, middle-aged with a large family, and Keri, young and single. Also during that time, Russell started kindergarten. We chose to send him to the Catholic school in town so that Christian values would be included in his education. As non-Catholics, we had to pay tuition, but we felt the cost would be worth the benefit for however long we could afford it.

In connection with our Moral Issues work, I attended a "Why Knock Rock?" seminar and brought back materials to share with our congregation. Also, after distributing copies of an essay I had written about the connection between Satanism and Halloween, I helped organize a family night at the church house on October 31 for anyone who didn't want to be at home during Trick-or-Treat hours.

Since we were still getting few visitors, Denny and I chose to invite someone over. We started with a new family at church, and we spent the evening playing table games and sharing our mutual faith. When the couple expressed an interest in getting together regularly to study the Scriptures, we invited them to come weekly. Soon another new couple asked to join us. Then others, including Darryl and his wife Katy, started coming. Before long, we had a full-fledged Bible study group meeting in our home. After feeling forgotten by our church friends, it was a blessing to have some coming over on a regular basis. In addition, a retired man named Ron Pelletier who visited shut-ins and nursing homes regularly began coming to see us. After a while, Denny started going to a nearby nursing home with Ron to minister to the residents.

After weeks of thought over my bathroom problem, an idea came to us. I could get my slacks up and down while dressing on my bed, so I needed to put that ability to use in the bathroom. I designed a padded bench just big enough to lie down on which would have a hole in it directly over the toilet. After getting my slacks down, I could sit up and position myself over the hole. One of the bathrooms was big enough to accommodate such a bench. The friend who had built the ramp in the garage agreed to make it and finished it in late November. Before I tried it, he said it should have a splash guard. We let him cut the bottom out of an old wastebasket and attach the basket as the splash guard.

The first time I used the bench I almost fell off because it was smaller and more firm than my bed. But with practice, using it became easy. It was wonderful going to the bathroom alone after two and a half years of needing assistance. The financial benefit of my independence was in cutting our hired help to eight hours per day. We now had Lois working from 7:00 a.m. to 3:00 p.m. five days a week and Keri two days. Since this left us alone in the evenings, we had Lois or Keri prepare our supper before leaving for the day and put it in the refrigerator. Between the three of us, we managed to get supper into and out of the oven or heat it on the stove, and I handled blending my portion. Washing the dishes at an ordinary sink from our wheelchairs was difficult, so we sometimes left them for Lois or Keri to do in the morning.

With our wage expense further reduced, an even larger surplus from each month's annuity check piled up in our bank account. We evaluated our living expenses again and noted the amount spent each month for rent and utilities. If we could build a rent-free, energy-efficient house, we could lower our housing costs. If we designed the house to meet our specific handicap needs, we might be able to cut workers' hours some more. At our current rate of savings, we estimated that by the time our lease on the Morley Road house ran out in June we would have enough money to pay for a small house minus the flooring. We had no problem with living in an almost-finished house since we had done it before, and it would only take a couple more months of annuity surpluses to pay for the flooring.

With cautious excitement, I drew a sketch of a floor plan I felt would work well for us, and we showed it to a builder. He wasn't sure we could build it with the amount we expected to have saved by summer, but it would be close. He agreed to do the job and said he would get back with us in the spring. Our future was looking brighter by the day.

Naturally, our lives were not problem-free. We still experienced times of sadness when we longed to be whole again. We missed physical activities like camping that we had enjoyed in bygone days, and I missed eating regular food. It was hard to discipline Russell when we were alone in the evenings, but we gradually learned how to correct bad behavior through loss of privileges.

Our biggest struggle was in our marriage. Denny's release from his past, my forgiveness of him, and our spiritual unity in dropping the lawsuit served to draw us closer together. This closeness was creating amorous feelings in Denny which he wanted to express through physical intimacy. I still found even the simplest attempts at closeness to be physically uncomfortable and emotionally painful and continued to reject his affectionate gestures. Moreover, I was afraid of getting pregnant even if we used contraceptives. I wasn't strong enough to carry a baby and give birth.

His feelings only grew more intense, however, as his deep need for affection, his near-normal physical strength, and our time spent alone together added fuel to his fire. He pressured me for sexual intimacy, and my repeated refusals made him increasingly frustrated. For the first time in our marriage, he said he felt angry enough to hit me. It was hard to see the strong bond between us growing weaker, and I felt responsible.

To make matters worse, two of the older Christian men that he often spent time with had told him a wife's duty is to meet her husband's needs. When Denny shared their comments with me, I was confused. Couldn't they see that I was handicapped, too? In fact, I was still about three steps behind him in physical progress. As far as I knew, they said nothing about a husband's duty to his wife. If they did, he never mentioned it.

I eventually gave in to him, believing the hurts I anticipated could not be worse than living with his anger. Our first clumsy encounter was an educational experience at best. We discovered that without touch Denny's body was sexually limited. He could not father children, and my fears of becoming pregnant dissipated. It did turn out to be as difficult for me as I had thought, but Denny felt better because at least we had tried. Afterward, an occasional rendezvous in his room whenever amorous feelings overcame him while we were alone became the new status quo.

(It was not the first time I had put his needs or desires ahead of mine. After Russell's birth, I had come under pressure to be intimate much sooner than my doctor had recommended. Worn down from a long labor, breast feeding, and a breast inflammation, I had been too weak to insist on having sufficient time to heal.)

We had not planned to cut back on hired help again before moving into the new house, but unforeseen circumstances changed our minds. One day in January Keri called in sick, and no one was available to fill in for her. We considered calling on one of our parents to help for the day but chose instead to spend the day alone. We made simple meals, washed all our dishes, and even managed to sponge bathe ourselves. We immediately set up a new schedule with Lois as our only attendant working an eight-hour shift on Sunday, Monday,

Wednesday, and Friday. She helped us shower on those days, and we did our own sponge baths the other three days.

With less help, Denny and I had to take on more of the chores. We made most of our meals when alone and also took on the laundry. Lois helped with it occasionally and also did the ironing. It was hard work, taking us twice as long as a normal person to do each task. But the more we did them the easier they became. The work served to improve our strength, coordination, and mobility little by little. Soon I followed Denny's lead and took the foot and arm rests off my wheelchair since they only got in my way. Sometimes we invented new ways to do old things. For instance, the potato masher gave us the extended reach we needed to press the fan and light switches on the range hood. Our limitations were challenging us to become more creative people.

With housework, church, Bible study, and getting Russell off to school by ourselves two days a week, we were becoming busy people again. Also, our determination to help the unborn was even greater now that Denny's past was out in the open, and our involvement in pro-life work increased. I called the headquarters of R.L.M. to arrange for one of their representatives to meet with us and several other local pro-lifers. We discussed the requirements for starting our own affiliate and officially created it in March.

Spring came quickly, and we talked to the builder again about the house. The additional cut in our wage expense back in January meant we would have enough money by summer for a slightly larger house, complete with flooring. By fall, we could afford to have a workroom and carport added on and asked the builder to include the addition in his fall schedule. But when we mentioned our plans to Kathryn, she generously offered to lend us the extra money needed to have everything built at one time. The construction was to begin in late May. Just prior to laying the foundation, the builder told us to mark the location of the house by driving a stake where we wanted its southeast corner to be.

On a warm May day, we went to our four acres and drove into the open field. After Lois unloaded us from the van, we scanned the gently sloping terrain and noted the location of the nearest utility pole. At Denny's direction, Lois paced off 100 feet north and 25 feet west from the pole and pounded the stake into the ground. Then we took a few minutes to bask in the moment. How quickly things had changed! We never imagined when we sent our letter to Todd that nine months later we would start building a new house.

I looked across the road at our old house on the farm. It had been three years since we had left there, but it felt like twenty years had gone by. Renters had moved into the house the previous year under Kathryn's supervision and with our approval. There was life on the farm again, and the abandoned look was gone. It didn't bother me very much anymore to be unable to live there. I guess I was just too excited about our new home.

Soon the construction began. The interior design of the house was crucial for ease of access and maneuverability. The doors and hallway needed to be wider, electrical outlets higher, kitchen counters lower, and three-way switches in strategic locations. The bathroom had to be big enough for my special bench over the toilet. Outside, there were to be no steps or ramps and lots of cement. Because the ground around the house needed to be level with the floor, sand and black dirt were hauled in and dozer work done. I had 101 ideas for making the house easier for us to work in, so Denny let me handle the interior planning. I lay awake nights thinking of time- and energy-saving ideas. I also chose the colors, carpets, and curtains. It was so much fun.

We went to the property often to see the progress on the house. Lois took us on her work days, and a retired neighbor, Bud Miller, volunteered to take us several other times. Sometimes Denny and Russell rode their bikes the two and a half miles to the property to watch the construction. After one visit to the house, Bud loaded us into the van, and then we sat for a moment staring at this incredible blessing. Denny turned and looked at me with wide eyes.

"Can we really afford this?!" he asked facetiously, pretending in front of Bud to be in over our heads.

"Yes, Denny, you know we can," I grinned.

Lois knew the new house would mean more independence for us and fewer hours for her and decided to find a different job. We understood, but it was hard to see her go. She had worked for us longer than anyone else—about 21 months. Once again we ran a "Help Wanted" ad, conducted interviews, and hired a new attendant. After just two weeks, she left for a full-time job elsewhere. Instead of interviewing again, we chose to hire as a temporary helper an 18-year-old girl from our congregation who had done some fill-in work for us. Though she had no nurse's aide training, Katrina was capable and handled the job well. Since Denny was able to shower alone by then, her only personal care task was to help me in the shower. Her job consisted mainly of housework and errand running.

The summer of 1988 was a hot one, and we were anxious to move into the new house with its heavy insulation, cool cement floor, and a ceiling fan in the great room. After two scorching months, the house was ready. We moved in on July 29 with the yard work still underway. The kitchen's low countertops, open spaces under the sink and cook top, and built-in oven at just the right height were perfect for our use in wheelchairs. Because of the bathroom's features, I was able to transfer onto the shower chair with my sliding board and shower by myself. With that accomplishment, Denny and I were both completely independent in our personal care.

Since Katrina was preparing to leave for college, we did interviews again and hired Kathy. With no help needed on personal care, nurse's aide training was not required. And with household chores easier to do by ourselves, we only needed to have Kathy work 20 hours a week. The reduction in wages and utilities plus the elimination of rent dropped our monthly expenditures by several hundred dollars and enabled us to cover all basic living expenses with our disability benefits alone. After paying Kathryn back the money she had lent us, the annuity checks were free and clear; we could use them for whatever purpose we chose.

The Lord's work in our situation had been nothing less than spectacular. Not only had he given us back more physical ability than the Rehab doctors thought possible, he had also brought us to a place of financial security and stability. We praised God for his goodness and took advantage of every opportunity to share our financial blessings with others. In addition, church groups occasionally asked us to share our story with them, usually in a Sunday morning service. God had turned an apparent tragedy into a triumphant story. He had indeed made all things work together for good.

Year: 2005

Dear Denny,

What a special time that was! Freedom for you from the past, acting on our convictions, receiving unimaginable blessings. We amazed the doctors, our loved ones, and ourselves. I want you to know how proud I am of you for being a man of faith and conviction. It was our finest hour together, and I will always be glad we shared that mountain top experience.

But a strange thing happened after we moved into the new house. Our rapid journey through the Land of the Impossible ground to a screeching halt. Have you ever realized that, Denny? The doctors had set the bar so low for our physical achievement that we couldn't accept it, so we pushed ourselves to go further until we were financially stable and sure our family would remain together. Then, we stopped. Why?

In my opinion, it was because we got bogged down in the quagmire of our own self-will. We kept on asking God for complete healing. But the unique house he gave us should have been a clue. Why would he have us build an accessible home if we weren't going to need it? Our resistance to fully accepting our handicaps was partly due to Darryl's beliefs about healing, but it was also because we thought it was the only way to solve our intimacy problem. (Of course, it wasn't.) I wonder how different our lives would have been from there on if we had accepted our handicaps completely. I wonder.

Love always,
Mae Jean

PART II

Hurricane

Chapter 6

Storm Clouds

Three years of suffering, uncertainty, and tough decisions were over, and our newfound stability appeared to be long-term. Ideas for making our wonderful new home even more accessible came to us from time to time. It had two bedrooms, one bathroom, a great room, and a workroom. We put Denny and Russell together in the larger bedroom, and I took the smaller one. We hoped that someday Denny and I would be able to share a room as most couples do and put Russell by himself, but that would have to wait.

Over the next two years, there were few changes in our lives, and those that did come our way were usually positive and by our choice. Kathy's work hours were reduced further as we handled more of the chores by ourselves. We also were receiving more volunteer help, especially with transportation. Family members and friends drove us to church services, get-togethers, and special events. They also helped us with outdoor projects.

Denny, the self-confessed dirt farmer, traded in the Honda Odyssey toward the purchase of a 26-horse Kubota tractor with a cab. He also bought a 13-horse Kubota and some implements. He and Russell raised a few vegetables for us and field corn for the deer and squirrels. Once or twice they raised a small field of sweet corn to sell and earned a little extra cash from it. Denny was fortunate that he had the strength and coordination to pull himself up onto the tractors. Attaching the implements was difficult, though, and often caused him great frustration. He wanted to be able to hook and unhook them by himself and not be dependent on others, but generally he needed help.

Denny also bought lots of power tools for his workroom. He had always loved working with wood and tried to find something he could make, given his limitations. He tried things like birdhouses and picture frames but never went very far with anything. He had some problems with coordination, of course, but getting sawdust all over really upset him. He got it on his wheelchair tires and tracked it into the rest of the house, which created more housework. The most serious problem, though, was the way the boards going through the table saw sometimes kicked back and hit him in the chest.

We did not discuss the possibility of contacting M.R.S. about vocational retraining again. We no longer had a financial need to become self-supporting. In addition, the M.R.S. representative's recommendation to move to Ann Arbor had obviously not been God's will since he had given us a personalized dwelling to live in right in our home area. We did not consider whether M.R.S. might have a Plan B for retraining and employment options closer to home.

Our boy Russell was getting bigger every day, and Denny bought him the kinds of things most boys want. First came the BB gun. This female, who had grown up in a household of daughters, tried hard to trust Denny's judgment about guns and boys. Next came a spur-of-the-moment purchase which was a little easier (and safer) to handle. One day Denny,

Storm Clouds

Russell, and their driver came home from town when I was doing something in my bedroom. Russell, carrying their latest purchase, came slowly and quietly down the hall and through my bedroom door. Immediately I saw it.

"What do you have there?" I asked softly.

"It's a puppy." His bundle of golden fur was pressed against his neck. I petted it gently, wondering whether I should be angry with Daddy for not consulting me.

"Well! Now you'll have to think of a name for him."

"Donny David," he replied without hesitation.

I tried not to laugh in his sincere little face. He had already named his golden retriever after the teenage boy on the dairy farm down the road. Housebreaking the puppy was a bit of a challenge working from wheelchairs, but Donny learned fast. Before we knew it, he was a 50-pound bundle of energy that loved to chase his tail, eat bugs, and have his back scratched. He turned out to be both a trial and a blessing in one hairy package. With Russell gone to school during the day, Denny and Donny spent a lot of time together and became best buddies.

We were glad that Russell was well adjusted despite the difficult years our family had been through. He did well in school and made friends easily. We had originally sent him to a Catholic school for his education, but after a year and a half we transferred him to a Baptist school. It was much farther away, and we had to carpool with other families to get him there. For the most part, the Baptist beliefs were closer to ours than Catholicism, so we felt the switch was an important one to make.

One of Russell's favorite people was Denny's friend Ben Talaga. Ben was a bachelor and a taxidermist several years older than Denny and was a little rough around the edges. The two of them had done a lot of hunting and fishing together over the years. Ben was pretty good at telling a hunting story and could be quite funny. One time the four of us were sitting at the kitchen table visiting when Ben got into one of his stories. Russell was laughing so hard at him that he slid off his chair and disappeared under the table.

Denny had three men who came regularly to get him out of the house. Ron still came weekly and took him to the nursing home to visit the residents. Bud liked to take Denny for a drive, to get a cup of coffee, or to visit someone. And then there was Ben. I was envious of these relationships and wished I had some women friends who could do the same for me as often as these men did it for him. The problem was lifestyle. Ron and Bud were retired, and Ben was self-employed with flexible hours. Most of my women friends had children at home, and some had jobs, too. They just didn't have much free time.

Another difference between Denny and me centered on parenting. Father and son were able to do more together than mother and son. They had biking, hobby farming, learning to shoot, assembling model airplanes, and quasi-wrestling on the living room floor. As a whole family, we had story time, movies, table games, and meals. But Russell and I didn't have anything that we did as a pair. Chances are, things would not have been much different if we had not been disabled simply because boys stick with their dads after a certain age. Unfortunately, we had no daughter for me to interact with.

As for community involvement, we maintained our connection with the pro-life movement and devoted as much time as we could to the work. As the local R.L.M. affiliate president, I did a lot of reading and information gathering, compiled a monthly newsletter, and led affiliate board meetings in our home. We circulated petitions, picketed abortion clinics, and attended R.L.M. meetings and conferences down state. We also had another request to share our personal story with other believers—this time at my parents' church.

Storm Clouds

Our Moral Issues directorship came to an end when we decided to leave our congregation and attend services elsewhere. The main reason for moving on was that we both felt the need for deeper spiritual teaching than we were getting. We had unanswered questions about how to cope with long-term limitations (especially in our marital relationship), and differing views about certain social and doctrinal issues played a part in our leaving.

Darryl's beliefs about healing were also prodding us to question what others in that congregation had been telling us and kept us striving to figure out what we were doing that was "holding up" our petitions for healing. Although Darryl's voice was the most influential, there were other people elsewhere making related statements. Once, we met an elderly pastor from a conservative church who made a much stronger statement. During his second or third visit to our home, my parents happened to come by. He made a comment to my father which shocked me.

"It's really too bad," he told Dad, "because if she just had enough faith, she could walk." I couldn't let that go by without answering for myself.

"I don't know how to have more faith than I already have," I told him. "I believe God can put me back on my feet in an instant if he wants to."

I shared the conversation with Darryl and told him the pastor had made me feel like a second-rate Christian. He was saddened by it and tried to encourage me. Darryl had never said we were lacking in faith. He had, however (perhaps unwittingly), implied that we were doing something that was causing the delay of our complete healing. On one occasion, he made a related comment about someone else. A member of the congregation had died of a chronic heart condition in his late 50's, and Darryl talked with Denny and me about his "premature" death.

"I don't understand it," he said. "The church prayed for his healing. I'll carry this to my grave."

After leaving the church we had attended for 11 years, we went to a Pentecostal church for several months where some acquaintances were regular attendees. It was a church with a strong emphasis on miracles and speaking in tongues. We never had a private discussion with the young pastor about our intimacy dilemma, but one Sunday after services I talked to him about the emptiness I felt during handshakes and hugs. He was not sympathetic. On the contrary, he thought I was being selfish to focus solely on what I personally couldn't feel during touching.

"Maybe you need to focus more on what the other person is getting out of the physical contact," he suggested.

Without knowing it, he was reinforcing the status quo in my physical relationship with Denny. Every time we came together, I tried to concentrate on the benefit it gave him and pushed aside my own needs. We were not sharing a mutually beneficial experience; I was simply allowing myself to be used. As the years passed, I felt less and less worthy of having my needs met.

We didn't find what we were searching for at that church and so moved on to another Pentecostal church where we had recently shared our story. Here, too, there was a strong emphasis on the supernatural. Although the pastor was young, we could see in him a deep commitment to seeking God's will and wisdom. During a one-on-one conversation with him, I brought up our ongoing struggle over intimacy. His comments were not helpful.

"I'm sure it doesn't make it any easier for Denny that you take good care of yourself," he told me. I thought, *What's that supposed to mean?* Was he implying that I should comb my hair less often or start wearing sloppy clothes?

Storm Clouds

Denny and I spoke with him together about it once. He understood that we were faced with a major problem. He promised to pray about it and get back with us soon. The next Sunday before services started he handed us a piece of paper containing his response. Hoping he had written something helpful, I read it immediately. He basically said that he didn't know what the answer was but quoted a Bible verse about being strong during trials. The bottom line was that we should not separate. If we did, it would hurt our Christian testimony.

My heart sank, and I felt the tears welling up in my eyes. I quickly asked Russell to take me out to our van. Once he had loaded me in and gone back into the church, I burst into heaving sobs. I knew our private battle was wearing me down, but it wasn't until then that I realized how desperate I was for some kind of solution. I felt so trapped in my circumstances with no acceptable way out. Denny knew my leaving was not a good sign, so he sent one of the older women out to the van with his jacket on the pretext that I might be chilly. She opened the van door and explained the jacket in her hand.

"Are you okay?" she asked with concern.

"Yes, I'm fine."

My lie was as obvious as my red nose, but she didn't press me to talk and went back into the church house. By the time the service was over, I was dry-eyed but exhausted. We went home and continued relating to each other in the same old way. What I didn't know at the time was that the storm clouds over the troubled waters of our marriage were slowly developing into a hurricane. It would eventually make landfall directly over my soul with the force of Frances and be more devastating than anything I had faced before.

What I did know was that people were always interested in hearing our story of triumph over tragedy. From our Rehab days onward, the idea of writing everything down in book form kept coming up. Once, while still living in the rented house, I sat at the typewriter and tried to begin a manuscript. I soon found myself putting too much emphasis on style and not enough on content. I didn't get very far.

In the spring of 1990, I decided to try again with a different approach. Instead of imitating the writing styles of other authors, I needed to develop my own style. The approach that worked for me was to write as though the people hearing the story were sitting with me and I was just talking to them. Nothing flowery or fancy or prize-winning; just keep it simple and tell the story.

This time the writing progressed well. I had no computer to work with, only my new word processing typewriter. Revisions meant retyping, which slowed me down quite a bit. After several weeks, however, I had to set the whole project aside because of emotional stress. The tension between Denny and me over our physical relationship intensified for no apparent reason. I felt too worn down and discouraged to write and told the Lord he would have to intervene if he wanted the book completed. Before long Denny announced that he was going to spend the summer living in our old house, which was not being rented out at the time. He felt he needed some time by himself.

Denny was able to travel from the new house to the old one using one of his tractors, the riding mower, or his three-wheeled bike. He had my dad carpet the stairs and then scaled them by going up backward sitting down. He would put his hands behind him on the next step and lift himself onto it while also pushing upward with his legs. He left his newer wheelchair behind and made use of his old chair in the other house. Less contact with each other meant less tension. I was soon feeling better and resumed my writing. For about three months he stayed there, visiting me often. It was summer, and Russell was free to sleep at whichever house he felt like.

Storm Clouds

Donny the dog was always with Denny. Late one evening when Denny was with me, we suddenly heard honking at the road. In the headlights of a car, we could see Donny's motionless body on the highway. We had let him out for a while, and he had tried to cross the road. The woman who honked was not the one who hit him, but being a dog lover she had stopped to help. She pulled him off the road for us and waited awhile to see what would happen.

After a few minutes, Donny struggled to his feet, ran in a circle, and fell down. Over and over he tried to walk but kept circling and falling. Kathryn came over and helped us tie him up in the workroom. He was not whimpering in pain, so we didn't call the veterinarian until morning. By then, Donny could stay on his feet and walk some. The vet, Ron Risley, who lived about a mile away, came to the house to look at him and told us the dent on the right side of his head was a crushed sinus cavity. The puncture wound on his shoulder caused him to limp badly but needed no treatment. Donny was lucky to be alive.

Through the summer months, my writing limited my involvement in our R.L.M. affiliate. Still, we had ongoing contact through our pro-life work with many people, including some area pastors. I spoke with one of them once about our marriage problem when he came to the house on affiliate business. He was sympathetic but had nothing helpful to offer. Denny and I together talked with yet another pastor, and he had no suggestions either.

From time to time we would discuss our problem with a friend or relative. Most were sympathetic but didn't know how to help. Occasionally, someone would lean toward Denny's overall needs being greater than mine. One of his relatives told me that being handicapped is harder on a man than it is on a woman, especially a man like Denny who was the outdoor type. Once again I sensed that he was being favored and allowances were being made for him. I wondered if she understood how difficult it was for me to be disabled. When we did discuss the nature of the problem with someone, we were careful not to be graphic. We were dealing with a very private matter. A generalized picture was the best we could give them. In any kind of physical interaction, the person who is the doer has more control than the receiver. During intimacy, Denny was in control and could easily adjust his movements if he experienced any discomfort due to our permanent sensitivity to pain and pressure. As the receiver, I had to explain any discomfort to him and hope he would make an adequate adjustment in order to minimize it. Additionally, there was the difference between the way men and women in general experience intimacy. For a man, it's mainly a physical act; for a woman, it's mainly an emotional experience.

Darryl was the person we called on the most for help, but he too was having a hard time counseling us on this one. There were plenty of Scripture verses about marriage, but how to apply them to our situation was another matter. He was sympathetic to both sides and knew we were trying to figure out a mutually acceptable solution that would follow Biblical teachings.

In one conversation, the possibility of professional counseling was brought up, but no one was comfortable with it. Darryl summed up our reservations well. He said it would take a counselor a long time to understand what we had been through and how our nerve loss affected us, and then it would take even longer for him/her to come up with a workable solution. It was better to continue working with someone who was close to us and knew our history. Unfortunately, that approach was getting us nowhere.

Sometime in late summer Denny moved back in with me, and in mid-fall I finished the manuscript. I concluded with a passage from the Bible which had become particularly

Storm Clouds

meaningful to me as a result of our experiences. "Consider it pure joy, my brothers, whenever you face trials of many kinds, because you know that the testing of your faith develops perseverance. Perseverance must finish its work so that you may be mature and complete, not lacking anything." (James 1:2-4)

At 112 pages, the manuscript was the biggest thing I had ever done on paper. I was so excited about it; Denny was, too. Throughout the writing process, I had shared each chapter with him as I finished it. We would read it together and then talk about it. Denny was encouraged by reading how God had been working throughout our ordeal. He was happy that his past could be shared so someone else in a similar position might find freedom like he had. Many times he was amazed at my recall. Things that he had forgotten became fresh in his memory again.

"I could tell you were writing everything down in your head," he told me, "the whole time we were in the hospital."

I wanted to get input on the manuscript from those who had been close to our situation. I had three photocopies of the manuscript made and started sharing them. The reviewers included my parents, Kathryn, Darryl and his wife Katy, Todd, and Dr. Palmer. Most of them were as excited about the book as we were. Three people, however, reacted differently. Dr. Palmer sent back a letter with the manuscript saying he still believed there was a possibility that our nerve damage had been due to the mushroom poisoning and not the Pyridoxine overdose. Todd chose not to make any comment or even return the manuscript. The strongest reaction came from Kathryn.

When I had given it to her and asked for her input, she seemed to be looking forward to reading it. When she brought it back, she said nothing about it and only spent a few minutes at our home, which was not like her. About six weeks passed without hearing from her, so Denny called to see how she was doing. That's when she admitted she was very upset over the manuscript.

For one thing, she thought I had been too critical of her care of Russell while we were in the hospital. The greater offense, though, was telling the world about Denny's past. She had been raised to believe that you don't air your dirty laundry. But Denny didn't see it that way. Sharing his past was a positive experience for him because he was free of the guilt and shame. Her views on spiritual things were often different from ours, and there was little chance we would ever be able to reconcile our differences on this issue.

When Christmas came, there was no family meal at Kathryn's house as usual, which we thought was odd. Some time later a friend told us he had seen Denny's family having dinner together in a restaurant at Christmas time. We put two and two together and realized that we had been left out of the family's Christmas gathering. Kathryn had been angry with one or both of us at times before, but nothing like this had ever happened. I had never intended to offend or hurt anyone with my book, only tell what God had done in our lives. Now we had to ask ourselves whether we should go ahead with publication. We decided to move forward while hoping she would cool off.

I contacted three publishers and got the same response from all of them. They were not taking manuscripts for personal stories and wouldn't even look at mine. They were interested in other categories of books. Denny and I then talked about publishing it ourselves since we still had some money left from the settlement. I contacted a printing company in a city about 70 miles away, and a representative named Russ came to see us. We learned that we could afford to have 5,000 copies printed.

Storm Clouds

One cost-cutting suggestion was to put the manuscript on a computer disk myself instead of paying the printing company to do it. Russ had contact with a woman in our area who published her own quilting books, and he thought she would let me use her computer for the task. When I talked to her, she not only said "yes", but she let me bring one of her computers home and taught me how to use it.

Kathryn's negative feelings about the book did not diminish with time as we had hoped. The anger she felt was shared often with Denny but never with me. She refused to speak to me about the book at all. She had always been a person who avoided direct confrontation whenever possible. She told Denny that if her real name appeared in the published version, she would sue me. We again asked ourselves if we should go ahead with the project. We both felt we needed to contact the other members of the family before making a decision.

I called Holly and Carl's house and spoke with Carl. I was shocked when he told me he had no intention of reading the book for himself.

"From what I've been told, Kathryn could sue the pants off you two," he said tensely.

"Carl! There's nothing in it to justify a lawsuit. If you would just read it, you would see—"

"I already told you, Mae, I am not going to read that book."

When I got off the phone, I was shaking. Later I called John and Sarah. Denny's brother John was a laid-back kind of a guy who rarely challenged or judged anybody's beliefs or actions. He didn't seem to be angry with me but said I should probably take their names out of the book, too. Sarah agreed to read it, so I sent her a copy. After finishing it, she told me by phone that it was not as bad as she had been told. She did, however, agree with Kathryn about my criticism of her care of Russell while we were in the hospital.

Denny and I prayed over the book, reread it, and discussed our options: Make no changes in it, revise it to suit his family, or shelf it altogether. We felt God wanted us to publish it without making any changes, and other reviewers did not feel we were hard on Kathryn in the book, so we pressed on. Once again we were making a life-changing decision and knew there might be painful consequences. I was grateful to Denny for being my book's biggest fan, even though it meant being at odds with his family. I was also grateful for his willingness to invest so much money in its printing. The shipment of my books was due to arrive at our house in late spring.

At the same time, we had to deal with another potentially life-changing event. For several months, Denny had been coping with the gradual enlargement of his left testicle. He loathed the thought of going to the doctor, knowing it probably meant surgery and who knew what else. He prayed alone, he prayed with me, and he prayed with Darryl that God would take the swelling away. Nevertheless, it kept growing. By late May, 1991, it was so large it had no place left to grow, and the pain was more than he could handle.

Right after the Memorial Day weekend, Denny had outpatient surgery to remove the testicle. While he was in recovery, the surgeon sat down with me and Bud, who had driven us to the hospital, and told us the testicle was cancerous. Denny was going to need a lymph node biopsy and chemotherapy. My reaction was minimal. After all we had been through, the idea of cancer made me think, *So what else is new?* Despite three years of relative calm, deep down I still expected our lives to be filled with drama and hardships.

Denny recovered quickly from the surgery, and his abdominal incision faded into a barely visible thin line. He was soon feeling strong enough to resume his usual activities. At his follow-up appointment with the surgeon, we were told that testicular cancer will usually metastasize, often to the

Storm Clouds

brain or lungs. Denny was told of the tests and treatment he needed next, but he said "no" to all of it. At first, the foreign-born surgeon thought Denny couldn't make out what he was saying because of his thick accent.

"Thees ees cansa. Do you undastand, *cansa*," he said a little louder.

"Yes, I understand that it's cancer," Denny replied. "You have relieved my pain, and I'm grateful for that. But I don't want anything more done."

"I am perturbed and disturbed," the surgeon said. He knew what would probably happen to Denny without further treatment. All he could do was send him a letter explaining again the seriousness of the diagnosis and waiving any responsibility for Denny's choice.

Some time later, Denny saw our family doctor for his second follow-up visit. The doctor told him of a friend from his college days who had been diagnosed with testicular cancer and died six months later. Still, Denny did not change his mind about getting treatment, and I did not pressure him to. Life with a major disability was not easy. I wasn't sure what choice I myself would have made if I had been the one with cancer.

In July, Denny's sister Holly reached her fortieth birthday, and Carl wanted to have a surprise party for her. Our entire household received an invitation and the offer of paid hotel accommodations so we would not have to make the round trip to Rochester in one day. We were encouraged by being included in this special event. When the day came, Denny was struggling emotionally over our issues and chose not to go. A woman friend drove Russell and me to Rochester and served as my helper when I needed to use the inaccessible bathrooms. I felt unsure of myself at the party because of the tension over my book. I didn't know a lot of people there but socialized as best I could. I noticed that Kathryn was not there and wondered why.

The next morning, we were invited to Carl and Holly's for breakfast before heading home. I had not seen or talked to Holly since the uproar over the book began. When I found myself alone with her for a few minutes on their deck, I cautiously broached the subject. I assured her that I had not intended to be mean with the book, as Kathryn had once told Russell, and encouraged Holly to read it for herself to make her own judgment.

"I don't want to because if I do I might find out that you're right," she said frankly and then added, "Whenever Mom talks about it, she just cries." As for Kathryn's refusal to discuss the book with me personally, Holly said simply, "If someone doesn't want to talk to you, there's nothing you can do."

In order to be supportive of her mother, Holly was denying the offending person the opportunity to share her side of the disagreement. If she had, Holly would have found herself caught in the middle. Unfortunately, the family's unwavering stand against the book was adding to my growing feelings of unworthiness. I had been a member of the family by marriage for 14 years and had had a fairly good relationship with everyone. Suddenly, I felt like I was not worth listening to. Kathryn's refusal to talk to me or include our branch of the family in holiday gatherings in her home was going unchallenged.

Year: 2005

Dear Holly,

Fourteen years have passed since that first Christmas I spent apart from all of you. Since then, I have been invited to your milestone events such as graduations and weddings but have not been included in gatherings of immediate family members only. Being ostracized was painful for me for years, but I have come to terms with it. Lately some small but positive indicators suggest that Kathryn may be ready to reestablish a relationship with me, but I don't believe it will ever be the same again.

I understand now how devoted you and John are to your mother. You will stand by her even when you know she might be wrong, even when it means that an in-law is treated like an outlaw. I would like to ask you a question, though. What were the chances that her conflict with me would resolve itself without your intervention? By refusing to look at both sides equally, you were not helping to resolve the conflict and therefore were contributing to the continuation of your mother's pain.

Sometimes I think it would have been in Kathryn's best interest if I had left all of your real names in the book because then she (with your support) might have gone ahead with a lawsuit against me. At least your lawyer would have looked at the evidence, and that might have led to a productive dialogue.

I still love you all,
Mae Jean

Chapter 7

The Pit

Denny's swift recovery from surgery was an indicator of his general health. He and I were healthy people—albeit, with neurological deficits—who didn't need to see a doctor any more often than the average person or take any medications. The development of cancer in his left testicle was predictable since it had been seriously damaged in a bike accident when he was a boy and had a lot of scar tissue attached to it.

Once he had recovered from the surgery, it was not surprising that he wanted to come together with me. We assumed the experience would be the same as before, but it wasn't. For the first time since becoming handicapped, he discovered that he had the potential to father a child again. The unexpected change made our intimate encounters more fulfilling for him and more frightening for me, contraceptives or no. I felt I had no other choice than to accept it and pray that God would help me through a pregnancy if it happened. I even tried to make myself happy about the possibility of having the second child we had always wanted.

In June we began distributing copies of my book from our home. At first, we charged $2.00 apiece to recuperate our costs, but after a while we just gave them away. We were financially blessed and wanted to give freely as it had been given to us. The response to the book was very positive. Many people said they were so captivated by it that they read it in one sitting. Usually, one aspect of the story was particularly interesting or thought-provoking to each person. Some kind of inspiration and/or insight was often gained.

The most amazing outcome from sharing our story was the contact it produced between Denny, Jake, and Anna. Jake told Denny she never had the abortion because she lost the baby spontaneously before the appointment. He could hardly believe it and asked Jake why he had not told him.

"I tried to, Denny," he said, "but you wouldn't listen."

Overwhelmed with shame at the time, he had not been able to discuss the pregnancy at all once he had given Anna the money and left. At Denny's request, Jake called Anna and got permission for Denny to talk with her personally about the miscarriage. She had left it to her brother to tell him and was quite upset to learn that he hadn't been able to. Nevertheless, finding out the truth brought even more relief to Denny over his past.

In spite of the joys and blessings of sharing the book, the emotional stress caused by the conflict with Denny's family, his cancer surgery, and the ongoing struggle over intimacy began to take a greater collective toll on me. I felt the need to lighten my load, and the easiest option was reducing my involvement in our local R.L.M. affiliate. I handed the leadership to someone else but continued to function as the group's secretary, compiling the monthly newsletter and handling some other paperwork.

Denny and I debated our marital dilemma excessively. Part of the problem was that we had too much time together and not enough meaningful activity for him. And the man could talk! One of his relatives and a couple of his friends admitted that he could talk things to death. Sometimes they told him to lighten up and be less intense about life. I lived with his intensity every day.

With or without a solution, life went on, and over the next year we made a variety of decisions regarding our lifestyle and Christian service. They were made partly out of a genuine desire to help others and/or become less worldly, but the underlying motive in too many of them was to please God so he would grant us healing. Besides wanting to be physically whole, we saw healing as the only way to end our battle over intimacy.

Sometime that year we left the second Pentecostal church and began attending services at a holiness church. Bud and his wife Jo Ann attended there, and we knew them to be humble, giving people. At their church, the people did not have TV's in their homes. The women did not cut their hair, they wore long dresses, and both men and women wore shirts with a sleeve length below the elbow. We also had met some Amish people who lived about ten miles away, and we occasionally spent time with them. They were even more conservative. They were also generous people and welcomed us warmly.

It wasn't long before we had our TV antenna taken down, and Denny gave it to his brother. We kept the TV and VCR for watching carefully selected videos. In addition, I decided to let my shoulder-length hair grow longer. I had read the passage in 1 Corinthians many times about women covering their heads with their long hair and had been leaning toward letting mine grow for some time. Being around people who believed in this practice made it easy to follow their example. Any other believers I had talked to over the years had said this teaching was no longer followed in most churches because it dealt with Bible-times customs and did not apply to us today, but they never gave me a satisfactory explanation of what that meant.

As our physical functioning around the house improved year by year, Kathy's work hours were reduced progressively, and she finally decided to move on. After that, we hired someone for two to four hours per week or accepted the volunteer help of a friend, if it was offered. Since our driving was being done entirely by volunteers, we sold the van and traveled in the driver's vehicle, which made the driver more at ease plus eliminated vehicle expenditures for us. We also began using the public transit system for going into town to run errands.

A couple of times someone suggested that maybe we had progressed enough physically to drive ourselves in a specialized vehicle. One friend with muscular dystrophy had recently had hand controls installed in her car and was doing well with that assistance. But Denny said it wouldn't work for us because of our limited hand-eye coordination.

"Ten miles an hour on the tractor is fast enough for me," he said. Since he was more capable physically than I was, I accepted his judgment and didn't think about whether I should try driving myself.

We had been giving financial support to the local Crisis Pregnancy Center but wanted to do more to help, so we volunteered to be a shepherding home—meaning, a family that takes in a pregnant woman whose crisis situation has put her in need of housing. During that year, we sheltered two women. The younger one was with us about a week and a half before she and Denny clashed over the housework. He felt she should be doing more light chores to earn her keep. But his tension toward me spilled over into one of his conversations with her, and he spoke harshly to her. A couple of days later she went to live with her grandmother.

The Pit

Later the CPC called and said a pregnant woman with a family was living in a leaky camper and needed housing for about a week until they could arrange for something better. We accepted the whole family—father, pregnant mother, two girls (ages seven and three), and a toddler boy. Their housing dreams were not realistic, and they stayed with us for six weeks before resigning themselves to a rented house paid for by welfare dollars. There was tension between Denny and this woman over their unrealistic goals. He was less vocal with the man, who was actually the one responsible for leading the family in an unproductive direction. Yet, Denny loved having the girls around, especially reading to them.

The most interesting member of their family to me was the clever three-year-old. One time she was playing in the living area of the great room while her mother and I talked in the kitchen/dining area. My back was to her, but Mommy saw her do something inappropriate and gently scolded her for it. Immediately the little one started to cry. Walking over to me, she rested her forehead against my upper arm, seeking comfort. Then suddenly she stopped crying, looked at her mother, and pointed at me.

"I love *her*," she said defiantly. I turned away momentarily so she wouldn't see my smile. Her always-calm mother just rolled her eyes.

"I can't wait 'til she's a teenager," she said in jest.

After their departure, our marriage issues just kept getting worse. For the second time, Denny became so angry during one of our debates that he said he felt like hitting me. I didn't understand why since I was giving him what he wanted—physically anyway. Emotionally, he was not getting what he wanted.

His reactions to my emotions and needs were varied and confusing. If he saw a tear slip from my eye during intimacy, he would say, "Oh, honey, don't cry." I knew he didn't want to hurt me. So to make this "necessary" act more positive for him, I would try to hide my feelings. The only way to successfully do that was to distance myself from the experience. I usually stared out the window and thought about something else until he was finished. Then he would get mad at me for being cold and withdrawn. I just couldn't win.

Occasionally someone would relate to us as if we were normal with just a simple balance problem. Denny himself did that with me in our physical relationship. One time while lying on the bed together, he touched me very lightly when my eyes were closed. When I opened them, I saw his hand and made a comment indicating that I had not been aware of the touching until I saw it. He shook his head in amazement.

"You look so normal!" he exclaimed, and I thought, *How can he not understand when he has the same condition?!*

"You have to accept that I have a handicap," I told him during one debate. "I can't be a normal wife to you anymore."

"Oh, but I do accept it," he insisted. His actions told me otherwise.

Another time I told him I was thinking about locking my bedroom door whenever I felt like I couldn't handle coming together.

"Don't bother," he said calmly. "I'll just kick it in."

He had never hit me, and I had no real fear that he would. Throwing or damaging a material object, however, was one way he occasionally used to vent his anger. While this is not an uncommon behavior among both men and women, his statement was not about venting frustration but rather about being in control. He was essentially saying, "You can't stop me from getting what I want." In spite of his calmness at the moment, I believed he would break open the door if I locked him out, and that did scare me. It made me feel even more trapped.

On many occasions, he said he would leave me if I ever refused to meet his need. He didn't say it as a threat but as an acknowledgment of his limits. He didn't think he could live with a wife he loved and desired if she refused him. I would always think back to other people's comments regarding his needs versus my needs: I was the stronger one; it was my duty to meet his needs; being handicapped was harder on him. I would especially focus on the one pastor's admonition to never separate. It appeared that I, the stronger one, would have to make whatever sacrifices were necessary to keep us together.

Darryl would sometimes mention Bible teaching videos that he found helpful in his own spiritual growth and lent us several of them. One contained a visual picture of unresolved issues that caught our attention. The Bible teacher drew a line on a chalkboard representing one's spiritual life starting at Point A, salvation, and working toward Point Z, spiritual maturity. Every letter along the way represented a point of growth. The Christian life should be linear, he said, always moving forward. If you find yourself circling in the same spot without advancing, it should be an alarm to you. God is trying to teach you something, and you're not getting it. You won't move forward spiritually until you do.

It was a perfect picture of our struggle. We were circling on the same issue year after year and getting nowhere. Our spiritual growth had come to a virtually standstill. With the lawsuit, we had circled for two years before finally taking that leap of faith which ultimately produced so much good in our lives. Although we knew we were circling again, the answer wasn't coming to us. And we were not sure who to turn to for help in finding it.

One night Denny had a dream which he believed was a message from God about our battle. It didn't provide the answer but showed us what was happening and was going to happen in the future. In the dream, Denny saw a man and a woman. The woman had a knife and used it to inflict a mortal wound on the man. Then Denny looked again and saw that it was the woman who lay dead on the ground. Not only had she been killed, but her body had been mutilated. Afterward, he felt something supernatural go through his being, a rush of power and peace like nothing he had ever experienced before. The dream ended with Denny saying excitedly, "Is this you, Lord?"

He told me about the dream and what he felt it meant. The woman was me, and I had wounded him when I kept refusing to meet his needs. But in the next part, I was receiving a much worse wounding at his hands. The ending indicated that one day there would be a tremendous peace for Denny. There was no indication as to my future. Denny's interpretation seemed logical, but it was ominous. Where would my wounding end?

By the summer of '92, we were becoming even more extreme in our self-scrutiny and withdrawal from anything we thought might be too worldly. We limited our video collection to only those movies having a Bible-centered theme. Even if they were clean and wholesome, they were not good enough, and we threw out movies like *The Lone Ranger* and *Bambi*. After a while, we gave up the TV and VCR altogether. The CPC had two counseling rooms but only one TV/VCR setup for showing informational videos to their clients, so we gave them ours for the second room. We were trying to root out any ungodliness in our lives, but no videos only gave us more quiet time together.

In July, we came to the conclusion that living on disability benefits was not God's will. We shouldn't be depending on the state for support but on the Lord, our families, and the body of Christ (the churches). We contacted the Social Security Administration and told them we wanted our benefit checks stopped. The representative convinced us to waive them instead of stopping them so we could reverse our decision if we chose to in the future. We also heeded his advice to continue accepting Russell's checks so that no one could claim he was not being taken care of. If we put the money in a savings account for him, it would be available for his needs in case no other funds came along.

If ever there was a time when we should have contacted M.R.S. again, it was that summer. Sadly, we did not view ourselves as capable of making further physical progress or finding employment. Our excessive focus on the intimacy issue was keeping us from trying anything new physically. We were spending ourselves on one thing and had no energy left for other pursuits.

Then in August we received what we thought was the answer to our prayers. A woman came to our door who had read my book and wanted to meet me. Her husband was with her, and we invited them in. Sharon was a young, quiet mother of two. After telling us how much she had enjoyed the book, she said she felt God wanted her to come to us to pray for our healing. She was from a Pentecostal church down state, and we were all ears.

Sharon, Denny, and I held hands while she prayed in tongues and then interpreted the message. God's word to us, according to Sharon, was that our physical healing was now beginning and would soon become evident a little more each day. When she left, we were practically in tears with excitement and wrote down every word she had said. We were so desperate for relief.

While we waited for the first signs of healing to appear, we carried on with life. We felt our decision to waive the disability benefits needed to be shared with others if there was any possibility that God would direct any of them to help provide for our financial needs. We drafted a letter and made copies for friends, relatives, and a few area churches letting them know the reason for our decision and Sharon's subsequent "message" from God.

Most people reacted to the letter either by saying nothing or wondering what was wrong with receiving government support in a case like ours. The greatest concern was expressed by my parents who were afraid we would only end up depleting our own resources. Only one relative and one friend supported the idea and gave us a little monetary assistance, but it was far less than we needed to live on. Yet, we did not waver.

That summer we also decided to home school Russell, who was going into the fifth grade and had asked to be home schooled. Some of our friends were doing it, it was cheaper than sending him to the Baptist school, and I had the skills. We chose to use the same curriculum as the private school just in case it didn't work out and we had to send him back. With so much to do, I resigned as the secretary of our R.L.M. affiliate. At the same time, the pastor who served as president needed to step down, and there was no one in a position to replace either one of us. Sadly, our group had to disband, and our members looked for other ways to contribute to the pro-life movement.

Home schooling was time consuming and required good organization. We had a schedule for daily school work and went on a few field trips with other home schooling families. I was glad that I finally had something I could do with my son. I soon learned where his strengths and weaknesses were. His favorite subject was History, and he was especially intrigued by the Pacific Theater of World War II. His hardest subject was English.

The biggest drawback to home schooling was the added work and stress. I carried all of the responsibility for it in addition to carrying primary responsibility around the house. Denny pitched in with household management and chores, but the only task he considered to be his alone was cleaning the linoleum floors. It would have helped if he had taken on more, like doing all the dishes, or he might have enjoyed working with Russell on one school subject. I never insisted that he carry more responsibility, though. I had learned to let him do whatever he felt comfortable with, and the rest was up to me.

Months went by without any sign of the healing Sharon had told us was in progress. Our intimacy battle raged on, and home schooling stretched me to the breaking point. I soon found myself breaking down over any little thing. I was under too much pressure. We called on Darryl even more frequently to discuss our problem. One time Denny drew a circle on paper and marked off his cycle of behavior in our relationship. First there would be an encounter, then a couple of days of guilt over hurting me again. Next came a few days of calm before he would begin to feel driven to have another encounter. I always agreed to it because I thought I had to, even if it meant stopping in the middle of some other activity to do it. Around and around the cycle went.

At some point, I began having drowning dreams. In each one, I was under water and struggling to reach the surface. I never made it. Instead, I would wake up with a start, my heart pounding, holding my breath. I would gulp in the air I had been unconsciously denying myself and lie awake for a while, trying to calm down. I had these dreams regularly for many months.

One day when I was feeling very stressed and overwhelmed, I went into my room to lie down and cry. Denny came in and sat near the foot of my bed in his wheelchair watching me sob uncontrollably.

"If this isn't a picture of mutilation, I don't know what is," he said sadly, referring to his dream. Still, nothing changed.

Knowing that I was having a hard time, three of my friends from our old congregation started making more time for me. They were Darryl's wife Katy, his sister Kelly, and a mutual friend Enid. Each one came to take me out of the house, sometimes even for an overnight stay at her home, whenever she had some free time. Their combined efforts were appreciated, and I tried to find some comfort in having time away from the stress once in a while.

The quest for godliness went on as well. In the fall, I had one of my Amish friends sew me two white head coverings. My hair was quite long by then, and I braided it down the side before putting on a covering. Denny loved to look at my long hair before I braided it each day. One morning when it was still hanging loosely over my shoulders, he sat close and admired it.

"I think God is getting you ready to present you to me as a new bride," he said. I smiled at him, but I felt sick inside. Did everything revolve around him?

In November, we made yet another church change. The vet, Ron, who lived a mile away, invited us to a Bible study held in his home on Sunday mornings. He referred to it as a house church, pointing out that the early believers did not have special buildings just for services but met in people's homes. Two Bible teachers came from a community to the northwest to lead the services on an alternating basis. Mike Steere, a man in his fifties, would teach for a month, and then Wes Beasley, who was in his forties, would come the next month.

There were other congregations that had the same approach to the Scriptures as this group, but they did not form a denomination. Each congregation was independent and there were no headquarters, but they had some joint ventures such as a summer camp for children. Some of their teachings were refreshingly different from what we were used to, and they were all grounded solidly in the Word of God.

Also in November a conversation with Darryl took a new turn. He could see how my emotional state was deteriorating, and he told Denny that he needed to leave me alone, as hard as that might be. Denny had great respect for Darryl and trusted his judgment. To my relief, he agreed to try it. I just hoped he would be able to do it.

For about three months we did not come together, but the tension in him caused by abstinence was hard to bear. One day in February he became so upset with me over it that he packed some clothes in a suitcase, called on his mother, and went to live with her. In a flash, we were separated (the one thing I could not allow to happen), and I was stunned. I called him the next day and asked him to come home. He was still upset and laid down two conditions for returning.

"Mae Jean, you have to stop crying over every little thing, and you have to stop insisting on having your own way."

His way or the highway. Think. Can't separate. What do I do. My mind raced, but I had no cards left to play and no energy left to fight. I told him he could do whatever he wanted if he came home. Kathryn brought him back, and in the evening we had one of our talks in my bedroom. This time there was no debate. There was nothing left to debate. He wanted to know if I meant what I had said over the phone. I suppressed all my emotions, remembering his two conditions, and gave him my answer.

"I meant what I said, Denny. You can do whatever you want from now on. It doesn't matter to me anymore," I said flatly. He smiled, turned his wheelchair toward the door, and reached for the door knob. Then he abruptly stopped and turned back to face me.

"Prove it by letting me be with you tonight," he said, pointing toward my bed. I pushed my feelings deeper. I couldn't afford to have any.

"Like I said, you can do whatever you want. Its up to you."

I did live up to my promise that night and committed emotional suicide in the process. My soul died as I gave up hope for any other way to keep my marriage together. To please my husband, I had to become an unfeeling shell, a possession kept available for his use. No solution had come from God in spite of all my pleas and efforts. Seeing myself as unworthy, I felt like God had abandoned me. I had never been so demoralized.

With the life drained out of me, my daily activities changed dramatically. I lay on my bed about 14 hours out of every 24. I didn't care about food and ate on the average two small meals a day, usually alone. I stopped home schooling my son and in its place spent hours crocheting alone in my bedroom. I no longer saw life in color, only in shades of gray and black.

Denny packed up Russell's textbooks and took him back to the Baptist school. When Darryl found out about it, he knew something must be terribly wrong and came right over. The three of us sat in the living room discussing what had transpired, including the promise I had to make in order to bring Denny home. Darryl listened closely to all I had to say, his face clouded with concern. He knew how deeply this had hurt me. Then he turned to Denny.

"And how are you doing?," he asked, apparently wondering how his friend felt about the pain he was inflicting.

"Oh, I'm fine," Denny said casually, missing the point completely. Darryl sighed and shook his head slightly.

"I could jump all over you for this," he said frankly. Then turning to me, he tried to offer some words of hope. It was useless, given the circumstances.

A few day later, Enid and I went to town and stopped at his office briefly. Darryl said he had been so upset with Denny during his visit that he had wanted to grab him by the shoulders, shake him good, and say, "Don't you realize what you're doing?!" I wondered why he hadn't and whether he would in the future.

Not long after Denny spent the night at Kathryn's, he got a call from her saying that John and his sons were coming up north for dinner. Did Denny and Russell want to join them? He said "yes", and the two of them spent a few hours there. But Denny returned home very distressed. When he had arrived at Kathryn's, he had discovered that the whole family was together. In other words, Denny and Russell had been included in a family-only gathering for the first time in a year and a half. I was the only one left out.

The curious thing was that there was no holiday. Denny assumed this had something to do with our marital problems. Now the whole family knew our marriage was in trouble, and suddenly he was welcomed back. At first, he had not spoken to any of them but eventually relented and joined in the family's conversations.

Denny was so torn inside. He wanted to be with his family but didn't like the shunning of his wife. He still loved me on a certain level and wanted to stand by me in the conflict over the book. But he wouldn't stop hurting me emotionally no matter how lifeless I became. His attitudes and actions were inconsistent and sent mixed messages.

We contacted Darryl less after the near-separation since there was really nothing left to discuss. In one of my phone calls to him, he struggled to understand why I had called at all.

"Is there something you want me to do?" he asked uncertainly.

I couldn't put my thoughts together very well at the time, let alone voice them. If I could have, I would have said, "Yes, Darryl, there is something I want you to do. I want you to protect me from my husband. You are the man he respects the most. If you don't hold him accountable for what he's doing to me, no one else will. Please don't abandon me, Darryl. I feel so alone."

About two months into my depression, I got an unexpected phone call that changed my whole perspective on our marriage problems. A woman in the next county had just read my book and wanted to tell me how much it had blessed her. Within five minutes, she turned the subject to abuse. She said that a woman who is being abused experiences a lowering of her self-esteem and a change in her perception of how God sees her.

"You just described *me*!," I told her in amazement.

I had always thought of abuse in physical terms or, on an emotional level, in the form of verbal abuse and belittlement. And Darryl had never described Denny's way of relating to me as abusive either. What I did understand was that I was useless to God. My whole existence had been reduced to trying in vain to meet Denny's needs and keep our family together. I had no joy, no purpose, no ministry, nothing. I opened my heart to the stranger on the phone and gleaned whatever help I could from her. She had just thrown a lifeline into the pit of my desolation and had given me a glimmer of hope.

When I told Katy about the stranger's help, she told me about a Christian psychologist in a nearby town. I made an appointment to see him, and she drove me to his office. The psychologist was an older man dressed in a business suit, and I was displeased that he talked more than he listened. His conclusion? I was obsessed with wanting to have a normal sexual relationship with my husband. *Me?* I thought. *No, I think it's my husband who's obsessed.* My hour ended, and Katy took me home. I never went back.

With the limited help I had gotten from the stranger, I determined that I needed to start standing up for myself in my marriage. I didn't know what kind of reaction I would get from Denny but knew I had to do something. I sat down with him at the table to talk about it.

"Denny, I have to start looking out for my own well-being because you aren't," I said nervously, trying to be brave. "I've waited a long time for you to change, but you haven't."

"You're right," he admitted humbly. "I haven't."

"So I think I need to set some limits. I need 24-hour notice if you want to get together so I can brace myself emotionally for it."

It was a cautious first step for a woman who had been yielding unconditionally, and he accepted my limit without question. I had finally gained a small measure of control, but at the same time I was losing something priceless. Since he showed no signs of changing on his own no matter how his behavior affected me, I didn't trust him. I could not look at him as my partner, someone with whom I could work toward a solution. Instead, I began looking at him as my adversary, someone from whom I had to protect myself.

My little act of self-assertion did not end the depression. People later told me I became progressively thinner and looked haggard during those months. I needed to do something more, but I wasn't sure what else I could do without making him angry. In June, my desperation drove me to a new method of seeking God's help. I told the Lord I was going to fast and pray until I was either delivered or dead. For five and a half days I consumed only milk, water, and juice. I prayed a lot and felt sure that an answer would come. Denny was surprised to see my energy increase somewhat during the fast. But half way through the sixth day I started vomiting. I had to either start eating again or keep vomiting, so I ended the fast. (So much for "delivered or dead".)

Just days later I told Darryl about it by phone, and he mentioned an upcoming prayer service at our old church intended specifically for the healing of human hurts. I hoped it would be the answer. Denny and I went to the service, and when it was our turn to be anointed and prayed for, the pastor asked Darryl to lead. Before the words came to him, he began to weep. I knew how badly he wanted physical healing for us. What I didn't know until later was that he had sensed almost immediately in his spirit that physical healing would not be granted to us that day. He prayed anyway, not knowing what God would do next. We left the service without an answer, and I remained desolate.

Over the next month, however, something did happen within me. It might have been due to the small control over physical contact I had insisted on or the warm weather or something spiritual going on inside or all of it in combination. But one day in mid-July I realized I was different. While sitting on the patio, I suddenly could see the sunshine and the leaves on the trees rustling in the breeze, and I could hear the birds' singing. In that moment, I knew I was out of the pit. It was like coming up out of a dark, suffocating hole in the ground and seeing life again. I was still perched precariously on the edge, but at least there was progress.

Year: 2005

Dear Russell,

You had such an unusual childhood. It certainly wasn't what your parents had planned for you. The physical disabling of your dad and me was just the beginning. It's a wonder you turned out so good. I think God blessed you in spite of us, our calamities, and our tumultuous marriage.

Although we never formally dedicated you to the Lord in a church service, we did dedicate you in our hearts, and that's what counts.

The most important thing we thought we could give you as parents (after faith) was a family that lived together under the same roof. We didn't think much about whether or how our marital strife might be affecting you. We probably thought we were keeping all the pain behind closed doors. But that wasn't possible, nor was it realistic to think we could. During my depression, I wasn't able to be much of a mother to you. I had sacrificed so much to keep your father with us, but the cost was too high. I lost my identity, my self-esteem, my joy, my purpose. It could be said that I wasn't really living in the same house with you and Dad; I was existing with you. You deserved to have a mother who was alive, self-confident, and able to nurture you.

Well! Aren't we glad those days are over? I hope God will allow me to make up for the years the locusts have eaten. At the very least, I want to become the kind of mother you deserve and the kind of woman you can admire.

Love you forever,
Mom

Chapter 8

Through New Eyes

A few weeks after sending Russell back to the Baptist school, he started getting sick on a regular basis. Our family doctor diagnosed his ailment as asthma. He was given a prescription for an inhaler to carry with him and use as needed. He missed a lot of school that spring and barely passed the second half of fifth grade. Years later I learned that asthma can sometimes be caused by stress. Russell had two stressors to deal with—his family situation and some boys at school who were bullying him. In August, I signed up for another try at home schooling. I was still not myself but was at least somewhat better, and Russell wanted to try again, too.

Knowing I was being abused, I looked at my options for counseling. There was a Christian counseling center about 70 miles away, but I didn't think I could ask anyone to drive me that far to get help. The other option was to counsel with Wes, who led Sunday services on an alternating basis with Mike. Wes had once spent several months in a wheelchair following the removal of a cyst from his spinal column. He had regained the ability to walk but was left with some permanent losses, such as numbness in the bottom of his feet. Wes had been counseling another woman in our congregation for a while, so I talked to her about him.

Rose Stone was a little younger than I and was married with three children. She had been meeting with Wes weekly for several months to work on relationship issues apart from her marriage, and he was helping her a lot. She had also read some books on her kind of issues and found Wes' approach to counseling to be consistent with general counseling practices. She gave me his phone number, and I gave him a call. He said he could start meeting with me on the same evening he met with Rose. Denny knew I was still struggling emotionally, but he had no interest in participating in the counseling.

"I've talked to enough people about this already," he told me.

He had resigned himself to our situation remaining as it was. I was the one who was willing to keep searching until I found the help we needed. Our marriage was unhealthy and had to change.

When Wes came the first time, I figured the best room in our house for having a private discussion was my bedroom. He stayed about an hour and a half, and I noticed right away how different he was from the psychologist I had seen. Wes listened almost the whole time, only speaking to ask clarifying questions as I related the history of our marriage problems, my depression, and the insight God had given me through the stranger. At the end, he spent a few minutes giving me some things to think about before his next visit.

The first few sessions were used to establish a rapport and helped me to become comfortable opening up to him little by little about my feelings, beliefs, and self-image. Denny never joined us, but he did strike up a conversation with Wes one time before we went into the bedroom to talk privately.

"I don't want to hurt her," Denny told him sincerely.

"Denny, I don't think you're the kind of person who would intentionally hurt anybody," Wes replied. "But I have to wonder how many more times this is going to happen before you stop."

Wes was so straightforward it amazed me. There was a lot about him that amazed me. He understood me better than anyone I had ever talked to. It was as if he could look right into my soul. He said he had once asked the Lord to help him see into the hearts of people, and God had obviously answered "yes". He wasn't claiming to be a mind reader. Rather, he understood human nature, hidden motives, and the effects of abuse better than most people. I only needed to say a sentence about myself in order for him to understand and verbalize a paragraph about me in response.

I talked with my friend Enid about the counseling and what I was gaining from it. Denny and I had known Enid since before the overdose, and she had watched our marriage deteriorate in recent years. Now she openly shared some of her observations with me.

"I watched you give up more and more of yourself," Enid said, "until it was as if you had become a non-person." Enid, like Wes, was helping me to look at myself through new eyes. In one conversation, she asked me a rather startling question.

"Are you being raped?" she asked bluntly.

"No. No, I can't call it rape because I'm agreeing to it." Then after a brief pause, I added, "But I don't want to."

"Isn't that the same thing?" she wondered. I told Wes about her question the next time he came to see me.

"Let's take out the word 'rape' with all the emotion that's attached to it," he suggested, "and let me ask you this: Can you say that you feel victimized?"

It only took a moment to admit that I did. I had never thought of my submission to Denny in those terms before. I had continued to agree to physical contact because I felt coerced, forced to choose between doing it to satisfy him or losing him and bearing the blame for breaking up the family.

"It's never right for one person to hurt another in order to get his own needs met," Wes told me in one session.

It wasn't long before the counseling started to get uncomfortable. Fortunately, the Lord gave me some dreams to help me along. In one dream I was in a large room with several other people, and we were being held captive. There was a door on the right hand wall, another on the left wall, and a window in the facing wall. Through the window I could see people who were free and enjoying the outdoors. A man took me to the door on the left and opened it. Behind it lay a dark tunnel and another door at the other end which I knew led to the outside.

"This is the way to freedom," the man explained. "But it will only work if you close this door behind you before you go through the tunnel and open the other door."

Wes and I talked about the significance of the dream. He thought the tunnel represented the dark, uncertain period I would have to pass through between closing the door on the abusive interactions I was still having with Denny and reaching the freedom God intended for me to have. I needed to make some painful choices without knowing what their long-term impact would be on our marriage.

Soon afterward, I realized that the counseling could only move forward if I became brutally honest about my emotional pain. That meant I might break down in front of Wes, which scared me to death. Crying in front of others had rarely led to comfort, and I had learned to push my feelings deep. During the five months of depression, I had almost never cried. On the day Wes was scheduled to visit next I couldn't do any school work with Russell because I was so anxious about what might happen during counseling. I told Wes at the outset of his visit that this might be a tough session, and then we began to talk as usual. I did fairly well until the conversation turned to the pain I had felt the night Denny had left me.

"At that point, you were essentially divorced," Wes commented.

"That's right!" I said firmly, feeling the emotions rising. "All of a sudden, you [Denny] were gone and I was alone!"

My voice broke, and I knew this was it. With everything I had in me, I forced my emotions back down, and my body reacted with disapproval. My breathing became shallow, my heart pounded, I was lightheaded, and my skin felt cold and clammy. Wes quickly moved his chair directly in front of me and laid his hand gently over mine. He spoke quietly and reassuringly to me, but I just couldn't let go. After several minutes, it became evident that I wouldn't be able to finish the session. Feeling shaken, I transferred onto my bed to rest, and Wes left. My heart rate and breathing soon returned to normal, but the cold, clammy feeling lasted for two days.

Before another session, Denny wanted to talk to Wes for the second time. That day he was feeling especially tense toward me, and he told Wes he just couldn't please me.

"Don't live to please her," Wes told him. "Live to please God and yourself." When Denny said he was, Wes expressed doubts, and Denny immediately broke off the conversation. His tension toward me began to spill over into his attitude toward my new counselor and friend. He could see a vast difference between how I responded to him and to Wes.

"You should see how you light up when you talk about him," Denny said once. *Of course I do*, I thought. Wes respected and valued me as a person, was full of wisdom and insight, endeavored to build me up (not wear me down), and was unquestionably God's answer to years of prayer.

It was hard for me to be as open about my feelings with my husband as I was with my counselor. One time I told Wes I felt so hurt by Denny that I wasn't sure if I still loved him.

"Now you need to tell that to Denny," Wes said.

"Oh! No, I couldn't do that. It would hurt his feelings."

"Mae Jean, you have to get over this fear of hurting other people."

It took me a while to realize what I was saying. I was so afraid of being accused of causing pain or hardship to Denny that I was willing to withhold the truth (which is a form of lying) if necessary. I was very confused and didn't know what a healthy relationship looked like.

During the weeks of counseling, Rose was eager to be supportive. She had been aware for a long time that I was struggling with something big. My sad countenance and hollow cheeks during the months of depression had spoken volumes to her discerning eyes. She admitted that she had wanted to talk to me and offer support during that period but could only stand by helplessly until I was ready to share my struggle with her.

"I wanted to help you, and I was mad at you because you wouldn't open up to me," she said in love one day. And I thought, *Now, this kind of anger I can live with.*

Rose and I shared frequently about our efforts to come to terms with our personal issues through counseling and reading relevant books. We became close friends, supporting and encouraging one another. The nature of our relationship problems were not the same, but we found common ground in the depth of our pain and in the changes we were being challenged to make in order to relate to others in a healthy way.

Denny and I continued to debate our problem often. One day he made a statement which gave me some insight.

"If only you didn't dress to kill," he said, looking me up and down. I couldn't believe my ears.

"No, Denny! I am not dressed to kill. I'm wearing modest clothes, and I am not dressed to kill!"

I looked down at my clothing—a long, full skirt and high-necked shirt in subdued colors, the same style I wore every day. And then there was my braided hair topped with an Amish covering. His ludicrous assertion opened my eyes like a slap in the face. I was not responsible for our marital strife, nor was I the one who needed to change. Wes agreed.

"All this time, Mae Jean, you have been looking and looking around your own life trying to figure out what you needed to do to fix this, and the whole time it was your husband who had the problem."

After about two months of counseling, I finally acknowledged that I didn't want to be touched by Denny at all. I told him there would be no more sexual encounters; they were just too difficult for me. Not surprisingly, he said he would have to leave. Soon he was established in our old house across the road. This time I saw the separation coming, I did not feel responsible, and I did nothing to try to stop him or bring him back. It was a painful experience, but I handled it fairly well. Home schooling went on without interruption. The living arrangement was the same as it had been during our brief separation years earlier. Denny came over to see me as often as he wanted to. He brought his laundry, we sometimes shared meals, and we handled practical matters, like finances, together.

My counseling with Wes went on, and many issues were addressed. When I told him about the years of praying for physical healing, Wes took a different view than others had in the past. In his opinion, it was okay to stop praying for healing and accept our losses as permanent. He was the first person to explicitly give me permission to be handicapped.

I stopped wondering what I needed to do to deserve healing and finally grieved for that which would never be regained. I stopped looking at the future in terms of when the healing might come and began instead to reshape my vision of the future based on reality.

There was also a growing emphasis on learning to feel freely both emotionally and physically. Wes and Rose were touch-oriented people, and I began to experiment with them on comfort touching. First, Wes started holding my hands through each counseling session. It was not done in the same way Denny had approached it. He would usually reach for and squeeze my hand in a spontaneous manner even though he couldn't feel either his hand or mine. Often he would inadvertently grip too firmly and/or press his fingernails into my palm causing pain unintentionally. In working with Wes, he and I simply laid our hands on top of one another in my lap. If Wes held my hands at all, it was very lightly done. Countless times, I stared at our hands as we talked, amazed that I could experience this kind of touching without feeling pain.

Next came hugging. Everyone knew Wes was a hugger, and he had offered to give me a hug soon after beginning the counseling. Now I started thinking about a way to tailor the experience to my unique needs. I suggested that he place his hands on my arms just above the elbows (a spot which was notoriously cold) so I could feel the warmth of his hands while I rested my forehead against his shoulder. The result was an experience in closeness similar to an embrace but with no pressure or pain. I shared this with Rose who gladly gave me a modified hug, too. Months before, she had offered to hug me, and I had turned her down because of my condition.

This simple beginning eventually led to more traditional (though still modified) hugs with them and with anyone willing to learn. One such person was my friend Cheryl. It was with Cheryl and her husband that we had begun the Bible study group when we were living in the rented house. The group meetings had later been moved to a different location, and we attended most of the time. Eventually, the group disbanded. We did maintain some contact with a few members, including Cheryl.

When I opened up to her about my marriage problems and the counseling, tears welled up in her eyes. She said she had always wanted to get closer to me as a friend. She learned quickly how to give special hugs. I called her from time to time for emotional support just as I did with Rose. One time Cheryl emphasized her commitment to me as a friend.

"If you need me, I'll be there for you in a heartbeat," she said. I was so thankful for another understanding friend.

Yet another dream made me think about my self-image. In it, I was holding a baby girl in my arms. She was about ten months old, completely naked, and sleeping peacefully. I stroked her soft skin and loved her as she slept. Rose thought the baby girl represented me and God was telling me to love myself as a new creature. I had been hard on myself for years while trying to live up to the expectations of others. It was time to learn how to love myself and rest. Wes and I thought her interpretation was right. Knowing it and doing it, however, were two different things. For a long time I was not consistent in following my heavenly Father's admonition.

I was still having a hard time connecting with the Lord after feeling abandoned by him during the depression. I asked Wes why he thought God had let things get so bad before sending help.

"Oh, Mae Jean, I can't answer that," he said. "You'll have to get that directly from the Father."

After praying about it, I sensed that it was because I had been relying so heavily on the judgment of people I knew well and trusted. Only a wound of that depth would make me admit they were wrong about certain things, turn away from them, and be open to a radically different approach. The two most important people had been Denny and Darryl, but they had plenty of less vocal or silently concurring partners.

One day in early January I spent a much longer time in prayer than usual. A lot of snow had fallen during the night, and I was alone in the house while Russell was out on the tractor plowing our driveway and a neighbor's. By the time I was finished, I had a greater sense of God's presence and love than ever before. When Wes came to see me a few days later, he noticed a difference in me right away.

"You look light," he said almost as soon as he sat down. I told him about my special prayer time, and he gave me a hug.

"This is what I live for," he whispered.

Not long after Denny moved out, he stopped attending services at Ron's house and switched to a congregation about three miles away. Naturally, the son followed the father, and I had to decide whether to make the switch with them. Since I had found what I had been searching for, I chose to stay put. I was gaining ground emotionally through Wes' counseling and growing spiritually through Wes and Mike's teaching on Sundays. And then there was Rosie. I looked forward to seeing her at services in addition to the one-on-one time she was giving me during the week. It was a hard decision, though, for it meant our family was divided on Sunday mornings.

One of the doctrinal issues I was paying close attention to was baptism. I learned that the word "baptism" literally means "immersion". There were many Bible verses connecting it to salvation and the putting on of Christ. Soon I told Wes that I wanted to be immersed even though I had been sprinkled as a teenager. At his church up north there was a baptistery, so we made arrangements to do it there.

Because of all the drowning dreams I had had plus my physical limitations, I was scared to be immersed but trusted the Lord to get me through it. I asked Rose if she and her husband Mike would do the baptizing, and she said they would be honored. During the previous months, a few of the men in our congregation had lifted me in and out of vehicles and carried me for short distances when necessary. Mike was the gentlest among them, making me feel very secure and comfortable in his arms. Rose was going to hold a handkerchief over my mouth and nose when he lowered me into the water. Since Ron wanted to be there, too, we considered his schedule along with everyone else's and settled on February 14, Valentine's Day. I had not chosen that date; the Lord had. I couldn't help wondering if he was trying to send me another message.

It was a very cold evening when Rose, Mike, Ron, and I traveled up north to meet Wes and his wife Alta at their church. The baptism took place without a drowning, and I came up out of the water relieved. Alta started singing "I belong to Jesus", and I saw Ron wiping the tears from his eyes with a handkerchief. It was a special moment.

I was doing better emotionally month by month but was still volatile. A quivering willow of insecurity, I was shaken by the slightest wind of change or challenge, doubting myself and others in spite of the gains I had made. One Sunday as Ron was driving me home from services, we talked briefly about the painful issues Rose and I were dealing with. He had a hard time relating because no one in either his family or his wife's family had faced anything like it. His conclusion, though, troubled me.

"Talk about being in the protective arms of Jesus," he said almost to himself as we pulled into my carport. Then he got out of his vehicle to get my wheelchair.

I sat there wondering if he realized the message he was sending. If the absence of problems indicated protection by the Lord, where did that leave us? Did our family's trials mean we were not protected? I had gotten the same impression from other people occasionally. I didn't know how to respond, so I said nothing. But his comment served to increase my self-doubts, and I again questioned my worthiness.

Another minor incident showed me how far I still had to go to heal emotionally. One day Rose told me that during Wes' last visit he said he was going to cut back their sessions to every other week. She was doing much better, and he thought she was strong enough to handle it. He had not told me about a cutback, so I assumed he would still come weekly to see me. When the next counseling day arrived and he did not show up, I was devastated. You would have thought he had broken a solemn vow based on my reaction. I called him, very upset, and asked him what was going on. Not telling me about the change was a simple oversight on his part, but he apologized for it. When he came the following week, he went even further.

"I accept responsibility for the pain you're feeling over this," he said.

Wow! I thought. *I've never had a man say THAT to me before.* My feelings over the incident gradually faded, but we could both see just how fragile I was. It took almost nothing to shake my sense of security and trust.

By that time, I was attached to Wes like white on rice. His unconditional love was just the beginning. Long before seeking counseling, I had lost the sense of partnership with Denny. Wes was now functioning as my new partner. He was someone with whom I could work toward the healing of my marriage. We had a common goal: Strengthen me so I could stand up for myself against Denny's abusive behavior and contribute to my marriage in a more honest, productive way. And Wes seemed to see a lot of good in this weak, pathetic woman. He once said he had high hopes for me.

Moreover, I was fascinated by Wes' life. He and Alta's first calling in the Lord's service was as missionaries. They had spent years overseas and were hoping to go back soon. He had all kinds of stories to tell, and I was an attentive audience. They spoke Spanish (the language I also had an interest in) plus a few more. For me, talking with Wes was emotionally nurturing, intellectually stimulating, and spiritually challenging. Then he and Alta started planning a six-week summer trip to China to teach English at a university. They asked all of us for support, which I looked forward to giving. But my enthusiasm for their work only served to increase Denny's jealousy of Wes.

"You might as well be his second wife and go to China with him," he said.

At the time, I thought he was being silly, but he was not too far off track. Wes had just given me another opportunity to partner with him (and Alta, too), so my view of him as a partner got even stronger. It was sad that my relationship with him did not produce a sense of curiosity in Denny. If he had looked closely, he would have seen what it was about Wes that made me light up and become engaged in life again. It would not have been hard for him to duplicate it and get the same response. My heart's desire was to feel just as safe, secure, and engaged with my own husband.

There were just two times when I questioned the closeness I had developed with Wes. Once, I wondered if the touching was really okay. This was unlike any previous friendship I had had. I did not share my doubt with him, though. I needed the comfort touching so badly and trusted Wes' judgment. On one other occasion, I wondered about the long-term prospects for our friendship. Wes had said he intended to be my friend for life. He was such an outgoing and loving person that I assumed he was just as intimate with lots of people. He had gotten really close to Rose, too. But I had to wonder how he could stay so connected to everyone he got close to over the years. Once again, I did not voice my doubt.

Despite Denny's negative feelings toward me, he never filed for legal separation or divorce. We were both committed to our marriage vows. We were just too opposite in our approach to resolving the conflict. (Wes once told Rose that watching Denny and me was like watching the Detroit Tigers competing against the Detroit Lions. We were not playing by the same rules.) I was also grateful to Denny for never using Russell as a pawn in our conflict. Russell had his school time with me and then was free to spend time with his dad. We never argued over our son or fought for his time.

Denny tried to reinforce his commitment to me by having our marriage license matted and framed to hang on the wall. I wasn't sure how to respond. When I told Wes about it, he noted the uncertainty in my voice.

"That was nice of Denny," he commented, "but it doesn't make you feel any more secure, does it?"

He was right. I had never doubted Denny's commitment to me. It was his manner of relating to me that had left me feeling insecure and afraid to get close to him. Nothing material could ever change that.

Denny eventually decided that living alone was too hard and said he wanted to move back in with Russell and me. Having seen no evidence of a change in his attitudes or behavior, I told him he would have to get counseling first. He resisted for a while before finally agreeing to it. Wes' trip to China was getting close, and he didn't want to take on marriage counseling. So a friend volunteered to drive us to the Christian counseling center 70 miles away, and we made weekly trips there for two months.

Our counselor was a woman about our age named Georgia. She viewed our problem in the same way that Wes did and focused on Denny's need to change. She encouraged him to lighten up our relationship by finding something fun we could do together. She thought he needed to court me again. He agreed to do it but never followed through.

During one session, the touching with Wes was brought up. Denny was against it, and Georgia saw it as questionable. At the counseling center, touching between counselors and clients was not allowed. I began to panic for fear that she would tell me I had to stop all physical contact with Wes. She had no idea how God had used him in my healing or how important comfort touching with this trustworthy man was to me, and my tears came to the surface. But she said nothing more about it and moved on to another subject.

Nevertheless, the pump had been primed. Some painful aspect of our marriage was brought up, and I began to cry. Over the previous months, I had been able to release some of my pain through tears when alone but never in the presence of others, not even Wes or Rose. Denny surprised me by showing compassion and started to move his wheelchair closer to me, but I wasn't even close to being ready to connect with him.

"I'm fine," I blatantly lied, trying to pull myself together as I held up one hand to him like a stop sign. We had so much work to do.

Soon afterward, my first full year of home schooling came to an end. Russell and I had gone all the way through sixth grade together, and the accomplishment made me feel good. It was nice to have the summer off for other things, but I looked forward to home schooling again in the fall.

As Wes and Alta's trip to China drew closer, his involvement in Sunday services ended. He was replaced by Bob Saxton, another man from up north in his late fifties. Bob was aware of our marital problems and came to see us one day. After visiting for a while, he offered to counsel us in our home at no charge as Wes had done with me. Denny was just beginning to admit his need to change and agreed to work with Bob. Although he respected Georgia, he said he probably needed a man to hold him accountable. I was encouraged, but I guarded my enthusiasm as we moved into this new phase of counseling.

Year: 2005

Dear Wes,

Thank you so much, my friend, for all you did to help in the healing of my heart so I could try again in my marriage. I understand that the Lord is the one responsible for my inner healing. Yet, he needed a willing servant to be his voice, his hands, his arms of love. You were the first one who was mature enough in Christ to know how to do that. Oh, there were plenty of Christians who loved me before you did. They just didn't know how to help.

It's interesting that God didn't send a woman to be my first and most influential counselor. He chose to use an honorable man to help me learn how to feel emotionally and touch physically so I could transfer the experience over to Denny and expand upon it. When I learned with you that hand holding and hugging could be comfortable and meaningful, I began to wonder what would happen in my sexual relationship with my husband if the same type of modifications were made. I also learned through you just how fragile my heart was and still is at times. I need to listen to my own spirit and set boundaries in all my relationships according to what I know I can handle.

There were some uncertain times in our friendship, but things have settled down now. I think our interactions over the past few years have been meaningful and mutually enriching. I'm so glad, but I must be careful not to hope for too much. I still miss you.

Siempre te querré,
Mae Jean

Chapter 9

Third Wave

While doing some cleaning and organizing around the house that summer, I came across a few books on Spanish that I had purchased years before. I had tried to study it by myself but had found it difficult to maintain my interest in it working alone. So I prayed over the books, asking the Lord to send someone I could either give the books to or who would help me study. A few weeks later I met Margaret. American-born, she had grown up in Peru as the daughter of missionaries and was married to a new pastor in our area. She was willing to work with me and began making weekly visits to our home.

About midsummer, Wes and Alta left for China. I missed him a lot but channeled my energy into letter writing and prayer support. I wrote every week and got almost as many responses in return. I had never been out of the United States, let alone to a communist country, and I thought they were so brave. When they returned home, I could hardly wait for them to come to our Sunday services to share about their trip.

They had slides and souvenirs to show and many stories of how they had seen God's hand in their work.

I was hoping Wes would start coming to see me again every two weeks, but he said I didn't need two counselors. He hadn't told me that before leaving. He probably assumed it was understood. I still couldn't handle unexpected losses well, so for the second time I was very upset with him. Wes and Alta made a special trip down to see me and tried to smooth things out, but the benefit was short lived. It was not just the unpleasant surprise that upset me. I was afraid of losing his friendship altogether if we didn't see each other with some regularity. Bob was a fine counselor, and we were building a good relationship. But the special bond I had with Wes could not be duplicated by Bob in such a short time. Wes had encouraged me to think of him as a friend for life without explaining exactly what that meant. Where was our friendship heading now?

There were only a few people who understood me, and I was afraid I couldn't be strong without having regular contact with each of them. I still lacked self-confidence. Without a lot of support, I didn't think I could hold up under the pressure from Denny and would slip back into the old ways of relating to him which had led to the depression. And I never wanted to go through that again.

I missed Wes so much I sometimes felt blinded by the pain. My friend Cheryl was going through a similar loss. She had never been close to her alcoholic father and had bonded with her fatherly pastor in recent years. Then he moved away, and she was beside herself with grief in the same way I was. I found some comfort in knowing I wasn't the only one. Rose had also lost Wes as a counselor and was trying to adjust.

In addition to changing counselors and beginning my study of Spanish with Margaret, another important change took place. Nothing good had come from waiving our disability benefits, so we had lifted the waiver earlier in the year. We had used up many of our reserves, including selling one tractor and most of the power tools. That summer we shifted our attention to opening a small business—a Christian book store—in the workroom. We used money from selling the other tractor to get the project off the ground.

The workroom needed some remodeling, such as taking out the wood stove and putting in carpeting. Then we acquired used shelving and other essentials from a store that was going out of business. Finally, we contacted a distributor of Christian materials to stock the shelves. It was only a small store (14' x 25') and we were located away from town, but we thought it was a feasible way to earn a little money without retraining or traveling. If it did well, we might even earn a living.

Although Denny was in favor of the idea, he did little to help get the store started. He had never been interested in paperwork and had always said, tongue in cheek, that he had married me so he would have his own private secretary for that sort of thing. Nevertheless, his lack of enthusiasm was due primarily to his inner struggles. He openly admitted limited engagement in planning the store.

"If it wasn't for you, this wouldn't be happening," he told me.

I hoped he would find the management of the store enjoyable, especially since it was Christ-centered and would help to keep us occupied year-round. The long Michigan winters were difficult for both of us because of our handicaps. We didn't go out much in the cold due to our sensitivity to temperature extremes, thus increasing our cabin fever.

Other, less significant changes had also been made. We called the Crisis Pregnancy Center to see if they were still using our TV and VCR, and they said "no". The center had moved to a new location with only one counseling room and our old equipment was sitting idle, so we asked if we could have it back. We did not put the TV antenna up again, but video entertainment helped to fill our spare time. We bought several wholesome movies for renting through the store and made sure we previewed them all.

It didn't take long for me to develop a close relationship with Bob, our new counselor. Several years older than Wes, he was more of a father figure to me. He was a hugger, too, but saw himself as less of an initiator than our mutual friend Wes. Denny seemed comfortable with Bob and came over to the new house consistently for our weekly sessions. Yet, he was not a person who was going to change quickly and continued to view our relationship in an unhealthy way. One day he made a stark confession to me.

"You are my drug," he said.

"No, Denny, I'm not a drug," I replied in frustration. "I'm a human being with feelings, and you can't keep relating to me this way."

It was the closest he ever came to admitting that he was abusing me. He knew he was using me in the same way that other people use drugs or alcohol to cover up some kind of inner pain. By then I understood why I had gone into the depression. He had sucked me dry emotionally trying to get his needs met and had left me too depleted to function normally. I needed to have my own emotional reservoir filled by him, but it had been a one-way flow of energy for far too long.

Control was a major issue for us. He still wanted to have it in our physical interactions, and I was terrified of giving him any. One day I was washing the dishes when he came up beside me to talk. He put his arm across my shoulder, and I became uneasy. I asked him to move his arm, but he left it there anyway, saying nothing. I asked him a second time, then a third, and got the same reaction. I looked directly at him and saw the determination in his eyes to do whatever he wanted.

With a small cry of exasperation mixed with panic, I moved my wheelchair away from the sink, which removed his arm from my shoulder. I moved backward about ten feet in order to put some space between us while I dried my hands and tried to regain my composure. I was easily panicked, especially by him. He moved a few feet toward me and then stopped. The look of contempt on his face was all too familiar. He spoke harshly to me as if I was the one with the problem, thus deepening my desire to stay away from him.

At Bob's next visit, I told him what had happened. Denny was remorseful over the incident, admitting that he had been wrong. Nevertheless, fresh damage had been done. Bob wanted to speak to us individually about it, starting with Denny. When it was my turn alone with him, Bob took my hands in his and gave me his advice.

"I told Denny that the trust factor here is zero," he said. "I think it's best if he doesn't come over more often than once a week for a while." Up to then, Denny had been free to come and go as he pleased. Bob's recommendation meant a first-of-its-kind visiting limitation, but Denny agreed to it.

For the first few months, the counseling with Bob produced only small improvements in Denny's attitude, and I would not let him move back in with me. Then a mishap called for a decision. One day in November I was using my bench over the toilet when suddenly I fell off. I had used it several times a day for many years without falling and couldn't figure out how it had happened. It was as if an unseen force had pushed me off, and I don't mean gravity. My knees were bruised, and the muscles in one arm were strained, making it more difficult for me to function around the house.

"Maybe this would be a good time to let Denny come home," Bob suggested. "There have been some changes in his attitude, and you could use his help. Maybe God wants to use this little injury for the good."

I understood his reasoning and agreed to let Denny move back in with me even though I was very nervous about whether we were ready for it. After his return, we remained abstinent but had many difficult conversations about it. Within a short time, I was feeling the increase in tension.

Then one night I had my first drowning dream in months. Fortunately, this one had a different ending. I was under water and desperate for air as in the others. The difference was that I managed to control my impulse to panic. I thought, *If I move my arms like this and my legs like that, I think I can get to the surface.* Soon my head broke through the surface of the water, and I took a long, refreshing breath of air. I did not awaken from this dream with a pounding heart and shortness of breath. The next day I understood its meaning. I was feeling emotionally overwhelmed again, but now I knew what to do to survive.

Bob continued his weekly visits, spending about an hour alone with Denny and the same with me. After a while, Denny backed away from the counseling. There were things Bob wanted to talk to him about, but he was not willing. There were issues from his childhood which Bob felt influenced his attitudes toward marriage, and there were Bible passages on marriage that they needed to study. Since Denny was unwilling to discuss these things, he dropped out of the counseling altogether. Bob and I maintained our counseling relationship for my sake. There was also the chance that the things I gleaned from him could be shared with Denny and he would still benefit from Bob's ongoing involvement.

In Denny's spiritual search, he made one last church move and went back to our old church, which meant having more contact with Darryl. Sometimes when he came home from services, he would tell me of a conversation he had had with Darryl after services were over. Even though Darryl had at one time been supportive of me, his comments now (translated by Denny) indicated disapproval of my recent choices. He questioned the abstinence, my touching with Wes and Bob, and some of the doctrinal issues that occasionally came up.

Concerned by the change, I called Darryl and asked him to come over to discuss some things. My preference was to talk privately with him, and he agreed to go into my bedroom/counseling room. He listened to everything I had to say and did not respond in a challenging or disapproving way, but he seemed more cautious than in the past.

At one point, we were looking back at the period of depression I had gone through, and he shared something I had not known before.

"I remember thinking I should send you flowers," he told me. "It stands out in my memory because I'm not a person who usually sends flowers. Did I ever do it?" he asked.

"No, you didn't," I replied.

Later, though, I remembered someone who *had* brought me flowers. Two older bachelor men in our congregation lived together and had a beautiful flower garden. Toward the end of my depression, their flowers began to bloom, and they brought me an arrangement every week for almost the entire summer. Each bouquet looked professionally arranged. When Darryl had not responded to God's prompting, the Lord had spoken to someone else's heart, and I had gotten more flowers than I ever could have hoped for.

Our little book store was not drawing much business, but it did provide some meaningful activity and contact with other believers. Financially, it was bringing in enough money to cover business expenses and pay our utilities. Denny was pleasantly surprised by his enjoyment of the store. He didn't mind the paperwork and handled the bulk of it for us. He especially liked going through the catalogs of new materials, reading some of the books we carried, and purchasing some items to give as gifts, usually to young girls we knew.

The tension between us, however, continued unabated. By early January, I was feeling too stressed by everything I was dealing with and knew something needed to go. I was home schooling, assisting some with the store, studying Spanish with Margaret, and counseling with Bob to cope with the marital tension. Russell felt ready to go back to the Baptist school, so at the end of the first semester we transferred him. This time I took him back myself and went over his schoolwork with his new teacher. We were using the same curriculum, and we were only a few days behind them. Russell adjusted to the change in no time.

For the next several months, no significant improvements occurred in our marriage. Letting go of home schooling didn't help it, and even the warm weather of summer didn't help it. Bob came to see me faithfully every week, and I made some progress as an individual. Denny was still battling inside over more than just abstinence, and there was no notable change in his view of me.

He was annoyed that I allowed Bob to hold my hands and hug me but refused to let him. He didn't understand my need to feel safe with someone in order to allow basic touching. As long as he didn't change, I saw him as a threat. The emotional wound was deep, and it was going to take more than abstinence to heal it. He did make an important observation one day after watching Bob and me share a farewell hug.

"That looked like it was very light," he said thoughtfully. I explained to him the importance of tailoring physical contact with me. Unfortunately, I didn't feel ready to give him the chance to try it.

Since Wes and Alta's return from the previous summer's trip, I had seen little of them. I called often to get emotional support from Wes, and he was always willing to give it. He and Alta were in the process of preparing for a full year in China teaching English through the English Language Institute—

China (ELIC). Much of their time was being spent traveling to familiar churches across the country that had supported their overseas work in the past as well as spending as much time as they could with their children and grandchildren before leaving. I still felt unsure of myself in the friendship since the unexpected loss the year before but wanted very much to support their work through letters, small packages, and prayers.

As summer drew to an end and the tension between us went on, I told Denny I didn't think I could face another winter cooped up together. If something didn't change for the better soon, he would have to move out again. But Denny refused to leave.

"I'm not going to move," he said firmly. "It's too hard living alone."

I then considered whether I could leave. There was no way I could get up the stairs of the other house, which meant I would have to rent a handicapped apartment in town. I would not be able to afford it on my disability check alone. So there was no way to get around being together for the coming winter.

After a year of studying Spanish with Margaret, we had to end our weekly meetings in late summer. She had registered for some courses at a nearby community college and wasn't going to have time for tutoring. I was excited for her but wondered what the Lord wanted me to do next. His answer came swiftly. The college was offering a Spanish course that was to meet at our local high school just five miles away. Some friends at our old church had signed up for it, including a middle-aged man named Ray Adams who lived two miles away. Ray told me he would provide my transportation if I took the course, so I registered for it, too.

From late August until mid-December, 1995, the conversational Spanish course helped to improve my speaking skills while at the same time giving Denny and me more time apart. The small class included four people from our old church. They had gone on a two-week missions trip to Ecuador earlier in the year and were planning to go back in early 1997. They asked me to go with them since my Spanish skills were greater than theirs.

I could hardly believe I was being invited to travel abroad and use my new skills in missionary work. Although I felt honored, I doubted that I could physically handle it. Soon, though, ideas for managing my physical needs while away from home flooded my mind. I felt like the Lord was saying, "You can do it. I'll help you." Denny was intrigued by the idea of going on the trip but was not interested in trying something like that himself. Yet, I had his blessing to go. With sweaty palms, I contacted the team leader, Dave Wolfe, and signed up. The trip was almost fifteen months away, so I had lots of time to prepare physically, spiritually, and linguistically.

When my Spanish course ended, I got an A, and I was very happy. Denny was proud of me and wanted to show it with a hug. He and I had been a little less tense toward each other lately, but some old habits remained. When I turned down his offer of a hug, he did not become angry with me as usual. Instead, I could see genuine hurt in his expression. I realized that I was letting my fear of closeness with him spoil an important opportunity. I immediately relented, and we shared our first mutually meaningful hug in years. Afterward, he went his way with a smile, and I sat there holding back the tears. I had done the right thing, but I was so scared.

Although we still had a lot of work to do in our relationship, we were making small strides here and there. We had reason to be hopeful, and we were by then in the middle of winter—typically our most difficult time of the year. But the battle was not over. In fact, a new phase was about to begin.

Third Wave

It started with pain in Denny's abdomen that worsened quickly. He saw our family doctor, who scheduled him for a gall bladder ultrasound. When it showed nothing, a surgeon scheduled him for a CT scan. On the films, two large tumors about the size of kidneys were clearly visible in his abdomen. At first, I was fascinated by the technology and how clearly the tumors could be seen. I didn't think much about what this meant for Denny, assuming that abdominal tumors could be easily removed. I was wrong.

The next step was a needle biopsy to find out what the tumors were made of. The result surprised us—metastatic testicular cancer. More than four and a half years had passed since his testicle had been removed. If this type of cancer was so aggressive, why had it taken so long for it to show up again? We didn't ask. We simply waited for the surgeon to tell us when the surgery would be.

As it turned out, immediate surgery was not an option. The surgeon explained that this type of tumor wraps itself around vital parts like blood vessels as it grows and is therefore impossible to remove. The prescribed treatment was intensive chemotherapy, then possibly radiation, then surgery to remove whatever might be left of the reduced tumors. The surgeon set up an appointment with an oncologist.

The cancer specialist did not have a good bedside manner. He told Denny what he would have to go through in order to be cured—three or four five-day hospitalizations for intensive chemotherapy two weeks apart with a single chemo injection half way between, then possibly radiation and/or surgery. He made sure Denny understood that he *would* follow instructions. If he had done as he had been told before, he might not be in such a predicament. (I thought the oncologist had missed his true calling in life as a drill sergeant.) The good news was that Denny had a 90 percent chance of survival. As much as he hated hospitals, he felt he had no choice but to give the treatment a try—for Russell's sake, if nothing else.

With the first hospitalization set for late March, Denny's family held a special family gathering for his March 9 birthday complete with gifts and a cake. Normally, they didn't get together for adult birthdays. The biggest surprise was that Kathryn included me. I had not been in her home in over five years, and I knew I was being included for Denny's sake. I was uncomfortable being there but tried to engage in light conversation.

When the hospital admission date arrived, a friend drove Denny to the U of M Medical Center in Ann Arbor and helped him get settled in. On the third day, he called to tell me that he was not doing well. The large doses of chemotherapy were taking a heavy toll.

"I don't think I can make it," he said. "But they tell me I can't leave."

Although he was having a hard time, the only way to be cured was to stay the course. He asked me to come visit him, so the next day Bob's wife Janice took me to Ann Arbor. Denny looked fairly good considering the circumstances, and I hoped our visit would cheer him up.

The next day was his final day of chemo, and another friend brought him home. He looked much worse and told me he had not been able to get into his wheelchair in the morning to go to the bathroom. The result was bowel incontinence in his bed. He was very weak but managed to get himself into our bathroom when needed. Perhaps being at home made it easier.

The hospital had made no arrangements for me to have help caring for him at home. At my insistence, they contacted the local Health Department, and a nurse was sent to check on Denny. She was very concerned by his weakness and his appearance. The color of his lips and other physical indicators signaled dehydration.

For the first three days, Denny stayed in his favorite chair, the tan recliner. I sat with him often, holding his weak hand in mine. Mostly he just looked at me and smiled, saying very little. In his current condition, he was no threat to me. I felt safe being close to him and wanted to help him in any way I could. There were many moments when I wondered if he would live through the week. Soon, though, he began to recover. His appearance and strength improved, and he slowly resumed normal activities.

Denny told me and all his visitors that he was not going back for any more treatment. Everyone knew what that would mean. I had to wonder just how difficult those five days of chemo had been on him. My mother was the most vocal in trying to dissuade him.

"But, Denny! If you don't go back, you won't get better!" she exclaimed. He just smiled at her, saying nothing.

Once he was feeling like himself again, we talked in detail about his hospital stay. When he had told the doctors on the third day that he wanted to go home, they had made him feel like he couldn't leave even if he wanted to. I expressed doubt over whether they could have forced him to stay. Apparently he had voiced the same doubt to them, and their response was shocking.

"Mae Jean, they told me that if I don't go back in two weeks for the next round, they'll send the state police after me."

My jaw dropped as I thought, *This can't be happening*. I asked him if he was sure he had heard them right, and he said "yes". He was determined never to go back.

"The chemo will kill me quicker than the cancer," he said.

He also told me about his last morning at U of M. In spite of his bowel accident, he wanted to get out of there. When the doctor checked to see how he was doing, he acted as though he was fine. Our friend/driver helped him into his wheelchair and out of the hospital. Denny was so weak he thought he was going to fall out of the chair but said nothing. He just prayed all the way to the car that God would keep him sitting upright.

The only positive news was that the tumors were significantly smaller. The doctor had told Denny he could feel a considerable reduction in their size through the abdominal wall. Nevertheless, Denny did not keep his appointment at the oncologist's office for his injection of chemo at the end of one week. The nurse called to find out why. I explained his decision and the reason for it, and she was deeply concerned.

At the two-week mark, he did not go to U of M for the next hospitalization. When one of the doctors called, Denny only spoke with him for a moment and then handed me the phone. I told him of the seriousness of Denny's condition on discharge and why he felt he couldn't handle any more treatment. The doctor was not aware of the bowel accident on the morning of discharge. I assumed it was recorded by the nurse in his chart, and he just hadn't checked.

"The average man who comes in here at 100 percent strength," he said, "usually leaves at about 80 percent, maybe 70." He seemed to be questioning the legitimacy of Denny's claim.

"But Denny's not an average man," I tried to explain. "He is strong but doesn't have the same stamina because of his handicap. He came out at 50 percent or less."

I also told him about Denny's fear that they would send the state police after him. The doctor was alarmed and said Denny had misunderstood completely.

"I was at his bedside when one of the other doctors talked to him about that," he explained. "What he told him is that we once had a state trooper in here for testicular cancer, and he was cured. A lot of these patients are in their early twenties. Now if one of them doesn't come back for subsequent hospitalizations, we send the trooper to their homes to *encourage* them to come in. He tells them he has been cured and they can be, too."

Well now, that made sense. I had to wonder if the doctor had shared this information with Denny in an unclear manner or if Denny's pain, mixed with his intense fear of hospitals, had caused him to hear it wrong. The doctor on the phone hoped that Denny would change his mind.

"We could try a lower dose," he offered. "The chance of curing him would drop, but even 80 or 70 percent would still be a good chance."

When I told him I didn't think Denny would return under any conditions, he was very disturbed. He knew their lack of sensitivity to Denny's unique needs was going to cost him his life.

When the phone call ended, I shared everything with Denny. Neither the explanation of the state trooper "threat" nor the offer of a lower dose made any difference. His decision was final, and I did not try to sway him. Only he knew what he could handle both physically and emotionally. He had been struggling with his handicap and related issues for eleven years. Life was a constant battle, and he was tired.

One of my aunts who thought highly of Denny called when she learned of his decision. She tried to convince me to convince him that he couldn't give up. He had to go on living for our son's sake. She was crying because she was so upset. Denny would not come to the phone to speak with her himself. The next day a letter from her for Denny arrived in the mail. If she couldn't get through to him by phone, she would try by mail. But her efforts were in vain.

As the weeks passed, Denny became his old self again except for the temporary loss of his hair due to the chemo.

We requested Hospice's assistance, and a nurse began weekly visits to keep track of his condition. An aide named Amy also came weekly for a couple of hours to help in any way we needed it—personal care for him, housework, or getting us out of the house for a while. We still had Bob coming to visit every week as well, offering any kind of support that either one of us wanted.

It didn't take long for our new reality to sink in. Denny's refusal to undergo any more treatment was a death sentence. He had not chosen to get cancer nor to have another bad hospital experience, but his decision meant certain death. This constituted our third wave of major trials—the medical mistake, the marriage conflicts, and now terminal cancer. Was life going to be one trial or tragedy after another?

Year: 2005
Dear Lord,
Your patience with frail humans like us is immeasurable. Thank you for never leaving or forsaking our family during all those turbulent, wearisome years. I looked at you as being harsh for a long time. Yet, slowly I have learned the truth in the expression, "Life is hard, but God is good."

The accounts in the Bible of people who suffered have helped me a lot. Job, for instance, was not stricken because he was bad; his suffering was not a punishment. Rather, you allowed Satan to test him to show how strong his faith was. When he challenged you, your answer was a scolding for talking back to you. I don't know why you allowed our family to go through so much, but I am sure you had a reason. If I really trust you, I don't need to know exactly what your purposes have been. I just need to keep trusting you and following your guidance one day at a time.

The trials certainly have produced a lot of growth in my life. Although each one left me depleted for a while, you always gave me the strength to carry on. I am a better person in many respects because of them. I cannot thank you enough for eventually bringing them to an end. If the only purposes for them were personal growth and the demonstration of your faithfulness, that would be enough. I have a feeling, though, that you want me to use my experiences to inspire and challenge others as well. May your will be done.

I trust you,
Mae Jean

Chapter 10

Lost Dreams

The five days of chemotherapy Denny had undergone at U of M had bought him some time. From his hospitalization in March until late summer, he experienced only minimal health problems. He worked in the bookstore, resumed his nursing home ministry with Ron, and took Russell fishing at a trout farm with Ben, the taxidermist. Nevertheless, there was a time bomb ticking in his body, and he knew it. Although we had made some small gains in our relationship, they were soon lost with the added stress caused by the cancer.

Denny still did not see how his behavior was keeping me at arm's length. His terminal condition made it hard for some of our closest friends to understand why I was not willing to get any closer to him. Bob, Rose and I knew it was a trust issue. I needed to feel safe with Denny first, no matter what he was facing. I had maintained contact with Wes in China by mail and occasionally by phone, and he also remained supportive of my position.

My friend Cheryl, though, found herself faced with a dilemma. Her little girl Jenna loved Denny and thought of him as her best friend. They would sit together in church, and he sometimes bought her small gifts. Cheryl knew about our marriage problems but now saw Denny primarily through Jenna's eyes. One day she brought her over for a visit. Little Jenna was happy to see that her friend was in good condition. The four of us sat in the living room and talked about a variety of things, including my trip to Ecuador scheduled for the following March. The Hospice nurse had told me to go ahead with my plans because Denny would not live that long. Besides, it gave us something positive to focus on. Denny remained supportive, and Russell eventually sign up to go, too.

Throughout the warm weather months, the Hospice aide Amy assisted us in our efforts to improve our relationship. I asked Denny if we could try going out to dinner, and he reluctantly agreed. He didn't like involving a third person as a driver on a "date", but we had no choice. Amy left us alone at Big Boy for about an hour to eat and talk. I still lived on a soft food diet because of the numbness in my mouth, but they had a broccoli soup I could handle. A second outing to Big Boy at a later time ended when Denny changed his mind in the parking lot.

One time when Amy took him out shopping, he bought me some new shirts. Only once when we were first married had he bought clothes for me. He and Amy came home from K-Mart with three oversized T-shirts in fluorescent orange, pink, and green. I had never worn anything like that. He said he thought they might brighten me up. His tone was critical, and the gesture lost its potential for good. I had no jeans to wear with them and they were much too big for me, so I had Amy return them. Over the previous year or so, I had in fact been buying brighter clothing, albeit in the same conservative style. The dull-colored skirts were slowly being replaced with corral and pink and purple.

In addition, I talked with Bob about my hair and covering. He gave me the first acceptable explanation of the Bible-times customs others had referred to regarding the passage in 1 Corinthians. It had to do with the way the temple prostitutes in Corinth had shaved or shorn their heads in connection with their idol worship. Then when they converted to Christianity, they tried to bring those customs into the church. Also, there was no sister passage in the New Testament, indicating that it was a problem specific to Corinth. I stopped wearing the covering and had about six inches cut off my waist-length hair. I continued to keep it braided or bound with a holder so it couldn't get in my line of vision and hinder my functioning.

I was facing more pressure from Denny with each passing week to resume sexual intimacy. One day Darryl's wife Katy dropped by unexpectedly when I happened to be in need of a friend to talk to about it. Katy listened for a while as I expressed my feelings, and she tried to be understanding. But something wasn't settling right with her. Then she told me why.

"It just seems cruel to deny something like this to a dying man," she said.

Katy didn't get it, and I didn't know how to explain it any better. In a phone call to Wes I shared her comment, and he was able to formulate a response better than I could.

"Mae Jean, that's like saying you should let Denny hit you with a baseball bat one more time for old times' sake," he said. "We're talking about something that's painful for you."

In August, Bob's wife Janice offered to take me up north to spend the night at their house and go to a women's retreat the next day. It sounded like a good opportunity for time away, so I accepted. Not long before that short trip, Darryl came over at Denny's request, and the three of us sat in the carport to talk. In this conversation, Darryl's disapproval of my choices was quite clear.

"I think you are hurting Denny as badly as he had hurt you," he told me.

Had he forgotten the depth of my depression? Denny was struggling with abstinence, but he was not in a pit, unable to function, like I had once been. His emotional state now was basically the same as it had been when we were coming together. He was not truly happy either way. The sexual debate was a symptom of a deeper problem.

"Darryl, I'm not against sex. But I have to see some sign that it would be different this time," I told him.

After a while I went into my bedroom for my usual afternoon rest while they carried on the conversation. When Darryl left, Denny came into my room to give me Darryl's assessment of me as a person.

"He says you have the spirit of Jezebel," Denny said. He seemed to agree with him.

I was horrified. Would Darryl really say such a thing about me? Jezebel, the wife of King Ahab in the Old Testament, was the most wicked woman in the entire Bible. To say I had the spirit of Jezebel was worse than calling me an unbeliever, a heathen. Darryl was saying I had an evil spirit in me that was bent on destroying the servant of God. The spiritual warfare was almost palpable.

It was no wonder that Denny and I were making no headway. His spiritual mentor was telling him the opposite of what mine were telling me. Bob and Wes thought the problem lay with him, and Darryl thought it lay with me. It was hard to fathom, though, because Denny and Darryl had both seen what had happened to me when we did things Denny's way.

I could not have been more relieved when Janice came to take me up north. Unfortunately, a day and a half was not a long enough break. I wanted to relax, but Darryl's bombshell had unnerved me. I returned home as tense as ever. Soon afterward, Denny began to experience more abdominal pain. The Hospice nurse worked with him on adjusting his medication until he was comfortable again. We anxiously waited to see if this was the beginning of the end. After a few weeks, he improved, and we carried on as before.

Soon I was feeling worn to the breaking point by the pressure to give in to Denny. Knowing how much he relied on Darryl for advice, I felt I needed to talk to Darryl again. I invited him over, and Katy came with him. His tenseness toward me was noticeable. He began asking questions which were perplexing to me: Why did I think I had to be in control of everything in our home? Had I been abused as a child? What did I expect from a red-blooded American male? I didn't know where this was coming from. I was only in control of the one thing that had previously hurt me so badly. I had not been "controlling" before Denny himself had abused me, and Darryl knew that. And I didn't know what his nationality and blood color had to do with it. I could only assume that Denny had been giving him a wrong impression about me whenever they talked.

Because I was emotionally exhausted plus confused by his line of questioning, my answers were too short, incomplete, and/or unacceptable. I felt hopeless and didn't see any good coming out of the exchange. After only a brief discussion, Darryl suddenly stood and turned to Katy.

"I have nothing more to say here," he told her. Then turning to Denny, he added, "I can't stay."

With that, he left the house to wait in the car for Katy. She stayed for a few minutes, telling us it was not a good week for Darryl to deal with something of this nature. She also restated her belief that it was cruel of me to deny my terminally ill husband what he wanted before he died.

Within days, I made the decision to yield. I just couldn't take the pressure anymore. If it had to happen, I wanted to be positive about it, so Amy took me to K-Mart to buy new sleepwear for the occasion and some contraceptives. In the evening when Denny came into my room and saw the new garment, he was overwhelmed. He was genuinely grateful to me for letting him do this and was extremely careful with me. He had never been so attentive to my physical needs. Although the encounter was not like they had been in our pre-handicap days, it was not painful. That in itself was a leap forward.

I was relieved and excited by the unexpected outcome. Not long afterward, I visited with Katy in their home and told her about it. She was very happy for us, and I knew she would pass the news on to Darryl. Sadly, however, Denny's new sensitivity to my needs didn't last long, and soon we were back to the old pre-abstinence approach. I did not withdraw from him, though, for I knew this would only last until the cancer got the better of him. But I went down emotionally again and battled daily to cope with our new arrangement.

Summer turned into fall, and Denny was still doing fairly well. He worked in the store and went to the nursing home with Ron. Amy came regularly as did one of the Hospice nurses, and I maintained my counseling relationship with Bob. Rose and my family provided unwavering support as well, and I knew my congregation was praying for us. But it occurred to me that I had not heard from Cheryl in months. One day I called her to see if everything was okay. To my dismay, all was not well in our friendship. When she had brought Jenna to visit Denny, she had thought I talked too much about my upcoming trip to Ecuador.

"I think you're too focused on your Spanish and your trip," she said. "It's like Denny's facing the cancer alone."

"Cheryl, I'm not going to die with him."

I tried to explain to her the need to have more than cancer in our future. Besides, I had his support for the trip. Yet, nothing I said to her made a difference. She never called or visited again. We had been so close for a while. Losing her at a time when I needed many supportive friends was quite a blow.

Denny and I carried on with occasional encounters to meet his needs. Sometime during the fall, there was one more time when he was sensitive to my needs, thus providing us both with a fairly positive experience. We were ebullient, but I tried not to get my hopes up too high. The next day we talked about it several times with smiles and a few tears. The second day Denny was still bringing it up repeatedly, and I told him we needed to move on to other subjects. By the third day his insistence on reliving it was giving me headache. He just wouldn't drop it.

"Denny, I'm glad we had a good experience," I told him. "But I don't want to talk about it any more for now, okay? I need a break, so I'm not going to discuss it with you for the next 24 hours." That made him angry, and we lost ground again.

When firearm deer season arrived, Denny, Russell, and Ben had their traditional hunters' breakfast early on Opening Day. It didn't take long for Ben to get a big buck. He had gotten only does for years and so was beaming with pride. We got out the camera and took a few photos of his trophy. Later, we gave Ben the negatives, and he provided us with two (yes, two) 8x10 framed pictures of him with his deer. We were glad to see him so happy, and I think the event brought some joy to Denny, too.

Within days of Ben's hunting success Denny's condition grew significantly worse. We moved him from the bedroom he had been sharing with Russell and put him in my room in a hospital bed. He had someone with him 24 hours a day.

Since Hospice could only provide full-time care once the patient appeared to be in his final days, Denny's male friends spent the nights with him. Men like Ron, Bud, and Ray took turns sitting up with him, taking care of any physical needs in addition to talking or reading the Bible to him or praying with him.

My temporary bedroom was the living area where I slept on the sofa bed. One night shortly after I had gone to sleep, I half awoke in a state of confusion. I looked up at the ceiling and couldn't tell if it was the ceiling, the wall, or the floor. I was thoroughly disoriented. Apparently, I let out a gasp or a cry, because I heard Denny's voice coming from my bedroom asking if I was okay. Momentarily, I was fully awake and oriented, so I assured him I was fine. This type of disorientation became a regular nighttime occurrence.

The Hospice workers expected Denny's condition to worsen any day. They thought he would be gone by Christmas, but he surprised them by improving around mid-December. The 24-hour help was canceled, and we resumed a fairly normal household routine. I found myself struggling with his recovery and talked to the Hospice social worker about my feelings. She said it was quite common in this type of situation for the family to actually be upset that the loved one didn't die. She said it was because I had braced myself for his death (which takes a lot of emotional energy) and then it didn't happen. I knew we would have to go through the same thing again at least one more time.

I didn't know whether to pray for his healing or for a quick death. My most frequent prayer ended up being, "Lord, do whatever you think is best." Denny naturally chose to pray for healing. He clung to Darryl's views on the issue, but I had let go. I still believed God could and sometimes did perform miracles but not with the frequency that these two men did. If the answer to believers' prayers for healing should always be "yes" as Darryl had once claimed, then God was a genie in a bottle granting our wishes instead of a sovereign Creator bringing his own plans to completion.

On one occasion, Denny asked Darryl to come over with some of the elders from the church to pray for him. After a few hours, Darryl showed up with two men in their twenties. None of the elders were available on short notice, so Darryl had called on younger men who were dedicated believers. The three men gathered around Denny in the living area of the great room to lay hands on him while I kept my distance in the kitchen area. As they took turns calling on the Lord, I was struck by one man's request. He asked the Lord to reveal any evil that the son might have brought into the home which could have caused Denny's cancer so we could remove it. I was silently furious. How dare he suggest that Russell could be responsible in any way for his father's terminal cancer. Denny did not challenge him on his request.

Christmas came so soon after his rebound that we didn't have much time to prepare. There was a hasty trip to town to buy gifts, but there was no meaning in it for me. I was too drained. Not long afterward, I realized how close I was to all-out depression again. Knowing I needed to let the emotions out, I went into my bedroom, closed the door, and muffled my sobs of desperation by holding a towel over my face so no one in the house would hear me.

One night I had my last drowning dream. It was quite different from those I had had in the past. I was in a car being driven by Russell. (He had turned fifteen in the fall and gotten his driving permit.) He missed a sharp curve in the road and drove right into a lake. The car sank, filling with water and trapping us inside. I gave no thought to Russell nor to how I might escape. I simply breathed in the water, hoping to die as quickly as possible. It was a disturbing dream, signaling to me that I was losing the survival instinct.

Through January, Denny was able to maintain his normal daily activities. We came together whenever he wanted to, but it gave him no satisfaction. He knew I was distant, and that frustrated him. Between his physical ups and downs and our marital roller coaster ride, I couldn't afford to take any more emotional risks with him. He didn't understand my needs in our sexual relationship nor in the battle with cancer, and I had stopped hoping he would.

One of the doctrinal issues we had disagreed on for some time was baptism. We had discussed it many times, but he was not interested in looking at specific verses about it with me or any of the men from the house church. Suddenly one day in January he told me he felt the Lord wanted him to be immersed. It was not the result of Bible study or a shift in his beliefs but was based on an inner sense. My excitement was guarded, knowing he might change his mind. I simply asked him where he intended to have it done and by whom. He chose to call on Bob. Days later, Bob immersed Denny in our bathtub with Ron Risley's help.

At the start of February, his condition deteriorated again with a tremendous increase in pain and the onset of vomiting. We reestablished 24-hour help for him with a variety of friends, male and female, volunteering to take turns day and night. Denny chose to stay in the living area on the sofa bed because he felt my bedroom was too confining and claustrophobic. Technically, I was his primary care giver. Even though I couldn't do much for him physically, I carried the responsibility for coordinating his care.

Denny and I had never liked taking medicine, and the Pyridoxine overdose had heightened our dislike. This was problematic for him, however, in managing his cancer pain. The Hospice nurses stressed to him the importance of taking the Morphine sooner rather than later so the pain wouldn't get out of control. Unfortunately, Denny often waited too long before taking it and suffered more than necessary as a result. In addition, he rarely took the sleeping pills offered to him, saying he wanted to be alert until the very end. Consequently, he was conscious of his suffering almost around the clock, getting little sleep.

More than three weeks passed with no change in his condition. Medication to alleviate the vomiting gave him little relief. He lost weight and became progressively weaker. I was feeling dazed by the ordeal, and other people saw it. Two Hospice workers said he was a demanding patient. One of them and Denny's friend Ron suggested that maybe I had done enough for him. It was time to let someone else carry the load. But Denny wanted to die at home with his family close by.

Then one night his mental state changed for the worse. Our friend Connie came to my bedroom in the wee hours of the morning and asked me to help her with him. He was desperate to get away from the pain, so we tried increasing the Morphine. Around 5:00 a.m. she came to my room for the second time.

"I'm sorry to bother you again," she said, "but he's trying to crawl to the door. He says he's going outside to freeze to death."

By the time I got into my wheelchair and reached him, he was close to the door. Connie and I talked softly to him, coaxing him back to bed. I called his primary Hospice nurse Terry, and she came over to work with him on pain management. A few hours later my sister Sue replaced Connie as my helper for the day. At one point, Terry and I conferred in my bedroom.

"How often do you have a patient who becomes suicidal?" I asked.

"Never," she said. "We're always able to control the patient's pain with medication."

While we were talking about our options, Sue knocked lightly on the door and then came in. She had tears in her eyes.

"He's heading for the gun cabinet," she told us.

Terry walked into the larger bedroom where the cabinet was located and casually asked Denny, who had summoned the strength to use his wheelchair, what he was doing. He became defensive, saying he just wanted to be left alone, but he returned to the great room without an argument. Terry followed and talked to him about being admitted to a hospital about 30 miles south of us for IV Morphine. He had sworn he would never go back into a hospital, but she was able to convince him that it was for the best.

Knowing the strain I was under, Terry suggested I go to a friend's house and leave everything to her. A couple from my congregation came over and took me to their home about three miles down the road. I rested in one of their bedrooms, wondering what was happening back home. After a while, I got a phone call informing me that the ambulance crew had just left with Denny. Before they took him out of the house on the stretcher, he pulled the keys to the gun cabinet out of his T-shirt pocket and handed them over.

Terry had promised Denny he would only need to stay in the hospital for a couple of days until his pain was under control. I went to see him the next day and found that he was easily agitated. I couldn't face having him come home and told Terry to let him know. She had previously told us about a Hospice facility an hour's drive away where she might be able to get him a bed. I was hopeful that he could go there—that is, until Denny himself called me.

"How can you do this to me?!" he demanded.

He had no idea how exhausted I was. Later a staff member at the hospital called me.

"Mrs. Mason," she said nervously, "it's his home, and we cannot tell him that he can't go back to his own home."

"Okay," I sighed heavily. "But if he has the right to come back, then I have the right to leave."

Knowing he was returning with an IV, I prepared the home front by putting Donny, the dog, in a nearby kennel. The risk that he would get close to Denny and pull the IV out with his tail or foot was too great. Then I contacted the parents of one of Russell's best friends and asked if he could stay with them for a while. He was also feeling stressed. When Denny returned by ambulance, Russell had not yet left, and I still needed to find someone to live with Denny as well as temporary lodging for myself.

Soon after his return, a medical worker showed up with all the IV supplies. He had papers for me to sign as the primary care giver and lots of medical instructions. A Hospice nurse was there, but he was addressing everything to me. I had no patience left for the unrealistic expectations of others.

"Why are you going over this with me?" I said angrily and pointed toward the nurse. "Tell her! She's the one who'll take care of the IV, not me."

Later that night his IV came out accidentally, and the nurse did not put it back in. His pain had diminished somewhat, and he was able to get acceptable relief from oral Morphine. We brought Donny home from the kennel since there was no longer any risk involved in having him around Denny.

The next day I told him of my intention to find someone else to be his care giver. On learning that Russell and I were both planning to leave, he realized he would die in his own home but without his wife and son around full-time. His mother had offered to take him into her home, so he called on her to be his new care giver. The Hospice nurse was concerned because of his mother's age, but his other relatives were willing to pitch in as well as the friends who had been helping me. Denny's family had been in close contact with us once his condition had begun to slip back in November. Most of them were understanding of the strain I was under. His mother, however, vacillated between understanding and criticism of me for not doing enough for him in his time of need.

Once Denny was settled in Kathryn's home, I went to see him every other day with the help of friends as drivers. During the first visit, I told him I was sorry I couldn't give him his wish to die at home. Still exhausted, I couldn't hold back the tears. He quickly summoned the strength to move to the edge of the bed to give me a hug. It was the only time in our 19½-year marriage that he had ever held me when I cried. A few days later he gave me a cross necklace that Amy had picked out at his request. I was touched by his gift, even though I knew I would only be able to wear it if someone else fastened the tiny clasp for me.

Amy noticed that he was a different patient after being moved. He was much less demanding in his mother's home. He expected less of her as an aide and less of his new primary care giver. He accepted fewer visitors each day. I took Russell to see him twice a week, but by the middle of the second week he wouldn't stay in the room with his dad for very long. Denny was so thin and didn't say much anymore. Bob said that for Russell the father he had known was already gone. Kathryn thought he should be made to sit with Denny after school every day, believing he would regret it when he was older if he didn't, but I never forced him.

Denny's condition became more critical with each passing day. His 44th birthday, March 9, came and went with no celebration. Whenever I visited him, I did most of the talking. He wanted to hear anything about life at home. My plans to visit him on Friday of the second week had to be canceled due to a snow storm. Amy told me by phone that the end was very near. His breathing was much more labored, requiring his oxygen to be turned up to the highest setting. He didn't want to wear any clothing, which Amy said was common with people who were near death. She was covering him with just a sheet. The next morning I called Kathryn around 9:30 to tell her we would be coming to see him in the early afternoon.

"Uh, Mae, someone will be calling you," she said.

Her tone was measured and somewhat businesslike. I guessed immediately that he had died in the night but did not press her for information. During the hour-long wait, I called Bob for support. Then Amy called and started talking to me as if I already knew.

"He's dead, isn't he," I said.

She was surprised that I had not been told. From this and later conversations, I learned that he had died around 12:15 a.m. while his brother was sitting up with him. He had been talking with John despite his labored breathing. John had turned for a moment to do something, and when he turned back, Denny was gone. He got his wish to be lucid right up to the last minute.

When I gave Russell the news, he sighed deeply and said, "Thank God it's over." I was both glad his suffering was over and relieved to be free from the pressure he had put on me over the years. Yet, I felt like half a person. The man to whom I had been committed for nearly two decades was dead. All hope of healing our marriage died with him. I wished we could talk one more time but knew it would not have made any difference if we could have. God had given us enough opportunities; time was not the issue.

I went to the funeral home later in the day to finalize the arrangements Denny had made the summer before. He had picked out his casket and his headstone, which he wanted inscribed with "Forgiven". (I wondered later how many people knew he had made that choice and not me.) Denny wanted the visitation to be held at the funeral home and the funeral service at our old church. He had asked Darryl to give the eulogy and had worked with Dave Wolfe, the leader of the missions team, on planning the overall service.

There were some small choices left to me. I went to a men's clothing store and picked out a light blue shirt for him (he always looked so good in blue) and a tie with dogs on it that looked like Donny. I purchased flowers, set framed pictures from Denny's life near the casket, and put a banner over it which read, "I go to prepare a place for Denny." At Russell's request, I got permission from the funeral home director to bring Donny to the visitation. A friend brought him for us half way through it, and they stayed about 15 minutes. Russell scooped up our dog in his arms like a calf so he could look into the casket.

The funeral went well with many friends and family in attendance. Denny was loved and admired by many for his faith and generosity. Several students and a couple of teachers from Russell's school came, too. As the mourners were filing past the casket for the last time, I saw Ben linger longer than most. When he turned to go, there were tears streaming down his cheeks. I held out my arm to him, and he came over for a hug. Days later he called to thank me.

"When I looked down at Denny," he told me, "I said to him, 'I'll see you in heaven.'" This rugged bachelor had just lost one of his closest friends.

After the internment, we went back to the church for the dinner prepared by the women members. When it was time to leave, I made a point of saying "good-bye" to Denny's sister, brother, and mother. Holly and John had remained supportive and understanding of me after Denny was moved to Kathryn's house, but Kathryn told Amy I had abandoned him. I don't think I could have ever done enough for her youngest son to win her approval.

Amy and another Hospice worker told me it was okay to be happy now. I wondered if they had seen a lot of new widows struggle to embrace life after the husband's death. I certainly had something big just around the corner to focus on. Throughout the year of the cancer, I had carried on with my plans for the missions trip to Ecuador, believing Hospice's prediction that Denny would not live until then. In fact, he lived to within seven days. We buried him three days later, which left Russell and me just four days to pack and secure the home before our first-ever international flight. It was as if the Lord was saying to us, "His life is over, but I still have work for you to do."

Year: 2005

Dear Denny,

It has been difficult but enlightening for me to write about our experiences together. I have relived all the pain but have also been reminded of the many times you and I were united in our beliefs and goals. You had many good qualities, Denny. You had great faith in the Lord and held staunchly to what you believed to be right. Your willingness to let me share our story through the first book has undoubtedly had a positive impact on the spiritual lives of many. Your nursing home ministry brought joy to the elderly, especially to Mrs. Montney. You taught our son about the Lord, hunting, gardening, even baking cinnamon rolls. And you remained committed to our marriage until death separated us. My emotional wounds have slowly healed, and I think you would be proud of the person I have become. My greatest concern is for Russell. Only time will tell how his views on marriage were affected by our conflict. I pray that God will provide him with a good marriage mentor before he takes a wife.

During the final months of your life, you reflected on your dream in which the man was wounded, the woman was mutilated, and you felt a great peace. You had wondered aloud if your impending death would fulfill the last part of the dream. I hope it has, Denny. Since you left this world, I believe you have been in paradise with the Lord experiencing the greatest joy and peace humans can ever know. Your battles are over, never to return.

Peace,
Mae Jean

PART III
Reconstruction

Chapter 11

Starting Over

Clothes. Check. Camera. Check. Spanish/English Bible and dictionary. Check. Nonperishable American food. Check. There were many things to pack for our trip to South America, but at last we were ready. Russell and I had gotten our passports and immunizations, we had arranged for Donny's care in our absence, and we had thanked God for giving us such an exciting opportunity so soon after losing Denny. Though physically and emotionally drained, I was anticipating a meaningful trip with a spiritual purpose.

On the morning of the big day, we got up at 5:00 a.m. and left home at 7:00. We met up with the other missions team members at the church in town and headed for Detroit. After a late breakfast at Cracker Barrel, we went to Detroit Metro and boarded our flight around noon. The first leg of the journey took us to Houston where we changed planes. The second took us as far as Panama. There, some passengers got off and others got on before we took to the air again. The final leg took us into Quito, the capital of Ecuador nestled in the Andes Mountains, around 11:00 p.m. I will never forget seeing three snowcapped mountain peaks shimmering in the moonlight above a cloud bank as we approached Quito.

We spent the night at the home of the resident missionaries, Kevin and Nancy, who were going to help us with the logistics of our trip. The next day was Sunday, and we attended church services in the home of an Ecuadorian family. After a fellowship meal together, I lay down in one of their bedrooms for a while. I was still very tired from the previous day's travels but was also feeling discouraged to the point of tears. Our enthusiastic leader, Dave, had altered our plans for the afternoon: Forego the full day of rest and travel to our final destination right away. About mid-afternoon, we boarded a bus bound for the coastal city of Esmeraldas.

At first, the bus ride was wonderful. The Andes Mountains were spectacular. After a while, though, the constant zigzagging on the mountain roads became more nauseating than the plane trip had been. And the driver was going awfully fast. I wondered if God was going to let the rest of our little family die as our bus tumbled down the side of one of those mountains. My anxiety eased after I told myself that the driver knew what he was doing and probably wanted to live as badly as I did.

The bus attendants served drinks and showed a movie on the TV/VCR to help pass the time. I had my own water bottle but drank very little. Too much would have meant asking other team members to carry me to the restroom at the back of the bus. After several hours, we left the mountains and drove for a long time through the coastal plains. By then, the word "torture" kept coming into my mind. At the end of six and a half hours, we finally reached our hotel in Esmeraldas. People started getting off the bus, but I had to wait for someone to carry me off. As Dave passed by, he looked down at me.

"You look like a cooked onion," he said with a smile and went on. *Thanks for the encouragement, Dave,* I thought wryly. In truth, I felt more like roadkill.

Our team waited outside the Aparte Hotel in the hot evening air while Kevin confirmed our room reservations. Once inside, we discovered that there was no elevator and no rooms on the first floor. Two men had to carry me in my wheelchair up to the second floor where I was to share a room with Russell. For a Third World hotel, the accommodations were good—a full-sized bed for him, a twin for me, an air conditioner, a small refrigerator with bottled drinks, and a private bathroom. Unfortunately, the bathroom doorway was not wide enough for my wheelchair to fit through. So the two other women on our team had to work with me on developing a way to get me into the tiny bathroom without the wheelchair.

The next day we traveled by taxi to our work site in a barrio called Codesa outside the city. A one-room bamboo-and-tin church house with a gravel floor was to be torn down by our men and replaced with a cement structure. We three women were to hold a Vacation Bible School in Spanish for the neighborhood children. The community was very poor, but the people were clean and friendly. It didn't take long to begin establishing warm relationships with them.

On the first day of work, half of the church was torn down while VBS was being held in the other half. We had just a handful of children, but they were already capturing our hearts. One little black girl named Jessica was about ten years old. She and her two younger brothers lived down the (nameless) street with their grandmother. Their mother lived in another province, and they rarely saw her. No mention was made of their father. Jessica wondered if we three American women could be her mother, and we had to blink back the tears. I wished I could take her home with me.

The second day's work included tearing down the rest of the church building, so the family across the street invited our VBS into their home. That day we held VBS indoors, but from the third day onward we met in their courtyard. We had more children every day in addition to some curious adults looking on. Because my Spanish skills were limited, I had tape recorded our Bible stories in advance. We had large pictures to show as each taped story was played. We also had a cassette of Bible songs in Spanish like "I'm in the Lord's Army". We taught hand gestures with many of them, and the children loved it. We handed out token gifts donated by church members such as candy and postcards, and one of our women had brought the materials for making salvation bracelets.

The men took some time off from their construction project to hand out Spanish New Testaments throughout the barrio. In addition, several of them had brought something special to share with the children. One had sports equipment, another had string tricks to teach them, and another had his guitar. The funniest of all were two men with nose flutes who had all of us laughing. Russell, being a bit shy, didn't spend much time with the children. But the señoritas would point at him, the only young and single man on the team, and say to me, "¡Guapo!" (Handsome!)

Occasionally, Kevin took us on an evening outing. We went to a local beach, to another one at the resort community of Atacamas, and to an open-air restaurant. We saw lots of scavenger dogs roaming around Esmeraldas and found the driving habits of Ecuadorians to be, shall we say, imaginative. According to Kevin, the posted speed limit in Ecuador was not a law but a suggestion. A driver only got a ticket if he/she caused an accident.

By the time we needed to leave, our men had done all the site preparations for the new church building and had poured the foundation and corner pillars. Some local men had

Starting Over

volunteered to help in the project as it progressed. Our team left enough money to pay for the rest of the work to be completed. The final total for the VBS was 70 people of all ages. We three women had done our work in a courtyard where the resident family of 14 was coming and going; plus, our men were in and out because they stored their tools, supplies, and personal belongings in the same courtyard. It was unlike any work environment most of us had been in before.

We were in Esmeraldas for ten days, including Easter Sunday. We had three days left—one for traveling back to Quito, one for tourism, and one for the return flight home. As we wrapped up our work in the barrio, there were many special moments and a lot of tears. The most poignant event for me was when the Ecuadorian architect who had been working with the men washed the dust from the wheels of my chair. He did it quietly and on his own initiative. It was like having him wash my feet. Despite the tears of almost everyone around me, I didn't cry. Having just come through such an emotional year, I did not allow myself to get too attached to anyone in the barrio. I wasn't ready to face another painful separation.

The return bus trip was divided in half. We traveled first to the town where Dave had led a missions team two years earlier. We saw the school they had worked on and shared lunch with the local pastor and his family. The second half of the trip took us through the mountains to Quito. Since our first bus ride, heavy rains had caused extensive mud slides. There were places where the mud had been cleared from the road with heavy equipment. In a couple of spots, half of the road was missing due to the mud slides, but we were able to get through on the one remaining lane.

After spending the night at Kevin and Nancy's, we discussed our tourism plans over breakfast. Originally, we were going to see the sites in Quito, but the new plan was to travel by bus for three hours (one way) to some Indian villages famous for their crafts. We had just taken one long bus ride, and I knew the next day would involve hours of air travel. I was too tired to spend another six hours on a bus in the mountains, so I wheeled myself into Kevin's office to cry. Soon I was found, and an adjustment in the schedule was made for me. Nancy would stay with me in Quito for local site seeing. Ray, who had helped me get to Spanish class, volunteered to stay with us. Nancy's three-year-old boy also remained with us while their six-year-old girl went with Kevin and the rest of the group to the villages.

Ray, Nancy, little Benjamin, and I went to a place called Mitad del Mundo (The Middle of the World), which was built on the equator. In front of the main building, there was a wide red line in the sidewalk representing zero degrees. Ray took a picture of me straddling the line with one foot in the northern hemisphere and the other in the southern hemisphere. There were many restaurants and shops there, and I bought all kinds of souvenirs. When we met up with the other team members for supper, we had fun telling each other of the things we had seen and showing off our treasures. As it turned out, Russell and I had purchased identical round llama skin rugs with panda bears on them.

The next morning we were up at 5:00 a.m. for a 9:00 flight. Our stop in Panama this time required everyone to get off the plane (except me) and take their carry-ons through Customs. The scheduled four-hour layover in Houston turned into a five-hour layover. We went on by plane to Detroit, by van to Pleasant Creek, and by car to our home. It was 3:00 a.m. when we got to bed; our 22-hour day had finally come to an end. I only slept for four hours, though, because I was eager to take my first shower in two weeks. Sponge baths in 100-degree weather were over.

Starting Over

It felt so good to be in our own home again with all its comforts, but we were glad we had gone on the missions trip. We had seen the mountains, experienced a different culture, helped to spread the Gospel, and pushed our limits. It felt like our lives had completely changed in a remarkably short time. Russell went back to school and I reopened the book store, but we were not the same. Our lives were not the same. God had a plan for the two of us which was just beginning to unfold.

During the next few weeks, I felt quite good. I was relieved that Denny's suffering was over and high from the trip. I spent a lot of time taking care of neglected tasks at home which had seemed unimportant while Denny was ill. Soon, though, the grief caused by being a widow at 39 sunk in. The emotions were a mixture of relief and sadness. Despite the joy from the trip, I became anxious about what God would allow to happen next. I didn't think I could face another major trial and begged God not to let anything as painful as the abuse and the cancer happen any time soon.

The frequent nighttime spells of disorientation I had been having turned into falling dreams, which lasted for many months. Each time I would half awaken and think I was falling off the bed. One time I must have screamed because Russell came to my room to ask if I was all right. Bob said these dreams meant I was feeling out of control.

Faithful Bob maintained his weekly visits to help me cope. He had been my shoulder to lean on for nearly three years. In addition, Rose and I often spent time together or spoke on the phone. Denny's friend Ron called me once a month to see how I was doing. He told me he had thought highly of both of us over the years, and he missed his ministry companion. He checked in with me regularly by phone for well over a year after Denny's death.

I didn't have much contact with Wes anymore but still missed him. He and Alta were finishing up their second year in China. Wes' responses to my frequent letters had ended after their first five or six months overseas. Alta took over their correspondence with me, but it wasn't the same. I had only met her a few times and didn't have the same connection with her as with him. Occasionally, I called China to talk with Wes directly. They had come home for two months the previous summer but couldn't spend much time with any one group of friends.

Our book store had been opened more for Denny's benefit than mine, so I asked the Lord whether he wanted me to keep it open. I tried to generate more business by sending out fliers to the area churches and regular customers telling them I would sell all merchandise at 10% off wholesale all the time. To my surprise, business actually dropped some. I took that as a sign and shifted to a going-out-of-business sale. By the end of June, the store was permanently closed. It took six more months to find another Christian book store to take my remaining inventory and all the store furnishings. Then Russell turned the large empty room into a home gym.

During the summer, I made use of some of the money left over from Denny's life insurance policy. Since he had left his job at the factory due to disability, his small policy there had remained in effect. After paying for the funeral, I had money left for minor homestead improvements, such as having gutters installed and paying someone to haul away some junk back by the woods. I also contacted Denny's brother John through Russell to see what he had done with our old TV antenna. He had no use for it himself and so had put it in storage. He brought it back to us, and Rose's husband Mike mounted it on the roof. It was 1997, but I saw President Clinton on television for the first time.

Starting Over

My long-term plans remained uncertain, so I asked the Lord for direction. For some months, I had given thought to the possibility of going back to college. Without Denny's disability checks, our household income was significantly lower. I had to consider the financial hardships I would face without finding employment, not to mention my need to be engaged in meaningful activity of some kind. Rose suggested I try becoming a Spanish teacher. I enjoyed Spanish and thought I might be able to handle teaching from a wheelchair. So in mid-August I took the public transit bus to the community college about 35 miles away to speak with an academic advisor.

I learned that I could transfer about a year's worth of credit hours from my two years of prior schooling. Then, after a year of study, I would have an Associates in Art and would need to transfer to a four-year institution for my teaching degree. The paperwork for financial aid was rushed through, and the cost of my tuition was quickly covered. I also went to see the M.R.S. representative to find out what kind of assistance I could get there. This time I was not approaching retraining from the same standpoint as in the past. The M.R.S. counselor was impressed that I already knew what I wanted to do and where I wanted to go to school.

My first semester required many adjustments—physical, emotional, and intellectual—which were to be expected for a recently widowed, just-turned-40, handicapped single mother who couldn't drive a car. The biggest physical obstacle was using the bathroom. On my very first day of college, I had to learn how to stand holding the handi-bar next to the toilet with just one hand while adjusting my clothing with the other hand. The first time I had to pray my way through the 15-minute knuckle-whitening experience. Eventually, I gained confidence and skill, making it possible to do it in half the time.

The changing of the seasons meant going out in the cold. Thermals under long skirts were not warm enough, so I switched to thermals under slacks. Transportation was provided mostly by friends who were also taking courses at the college. Occasionally, I had to call on my Spanish teacher, Russell, or the transit system.

Academically, I handled the course work well and consistently got high marks. But my anxiety over grades made it hard to enjoy my success. I spoke with two of my professors about it. One agreed that a high GPA in college would give me an edge someday when competing for jobs against non-handicapped applicants. The other, however, cautioned me about setting my standard too high. If I got straight A's, people would expect that kind of performance from me all the time. Too much of my self-worth was tied to my performance, so I persisted in my intense devotion to my schoolwork. Nevertheless, I did find some enjoyment in my new project. There were interesting people to meet, things to learn, and things to do.

An even deeper subconscious anxiety came to light through a revealing dream. In it, I was standing several feet from Denny's casket. Suddenly, his eyes fluttered open and he stood up. I observed him for a moment and thought carefully about how I should respond to his return from the dead. I knew that only God could raise the dead and I had to accept this as being his will. I approached Denny cautiously to speak to him.

"Denny, you need to know that a lot has changed since you've been gone. I've gone back to college, and I'm not going to quit."

When I shared my dream with Bob, he said I had an unconscious fear that Denny would come back. Deep down I felt he had held me back, and I was afraid of having to face that again. In truth, he had kept himself from advancing, too.

God only knows how different our lives would have been if we had both resolved the issues of physical restoration and marital intimacy.

I was still struggling emotionally over many things. My self-esteem remained low due to all the years of personal challenges in my marriage and in other relationships. I doubted almost every decision I made and couldn't grasp the significance of the blessings God was sending my way. Russell was well adjusted and a good son, but I felt the pressure of being a single mother. Although I knew I could remarry, I expected to remain a widow until I died. And I continued to deal with the day-to-day hardships inherent with a major handicap and the stress of being a middle-aged college student.

Yet, there was no doubt that God was doing a new thing in me and was blessing my efforts. Sometimes I thought he was expecting me to move forward too rapidly. I asked him why he wanted me to go so fast and sensed that we were making up for lost time. I should have and could have gotten retraining years earlier. Although I understood this and wanted to have a better life, I did my share of complaining about it. God was leading me into a new life, all right; but he had to lead me by the ear, kicking and screaming.

I hungered for more emotional support than I was getting. No matter how hard Bob and Rose worked to give me all they could, I wanted more from family, friends, and church members. Occasionally, I tried to ask for it, but my requests produced very little. I may have been too timid in my asking, or others might not have responded because they were too busy, didn't understand the need, or thought it was someone else's responsibility. During the fall, I started attending services at our old church with Russell. I thought it would be good for us to be together on Sundays and hoped I might meet some more people there who would be able to minister to my need. I wasn't looking for better Bible teaching; I was getting great teaching in the house church. The change did not alter my relationships with Bob and Rose in any way.

In December, I finished my first semester of college with a 4.0 GPA, which lifted my spirits for a while. After a long Christmas break, I went into the second semester with the same intensity and anxiety as the first. Once again, I came through with all A's. The semester ended in early May, and I had several weeks off before the start of my summer course, which would be my last at the community college.

During that time, I took care of some family matters. The car that Russell (now 16 and licensed) had been driving was an old station wagon that some friends had given to us while Denny was still alive. We went to a local car dealership and traded it in on a late-model Sundance. It was more fun for Russell to drive and burned less gas on his long weekday commute to the Baptist school. Also during my time off, I worked with one of my sisters and my parents on resolving a serious conflict in their relationship. I had been aware of it for a long time but wasn't in a position to be of help until some of my own issues had diminished somewhat.

One day I got a surprise phone call from the editor of *World Mission People* magazine. One of the men from our missions team had written several articles for the magazine about his various missions trips, including one about our trip to Ecuador. When the editor heard about me, he wanted to know more about the short-term missionary in a wheelchair. He asked me to write my own article. Of course I said "yes". In it, I described the circumstances Russell and I faced before leaving the country, the extent of my handicap, and the highlights from our two weeks abroad. The article was published at the end of the year.

While still attending the community college, I began to look at four-year institutions. I was willing to relocate, but the Lord was not leading me to do so. The closest university was

Saginaw Valley State University 60 miles away. Many middle-aged people in our area who went back to college commuted to SVSU. Some young people preferred commuting over living on campus as well. I went to the university and made the arrangements for the transfer without knowing how I was going to get there. The Lord was faithful and provided people for me to ride with by the time classes began in the fall.

My plans to become certified in Secondary Education meant I needed to choose a minor to go with my Spanish major, and I settled on French. The instructor for my first Spanish course at SVSU was the Columbian-born director of the Bilingual Education Program, Dr. Gladys Hernández-VonHoff. Just a few weeks into the course, she asked me if I would consider joining the program. She thought my Spanish was good, and there were financial benefits to being in the program. So I took the entrance exam and signed on.

In the middle of my second year of college, Russell asked my permission to go on another missions trip. It was especially for teens and was being organized by the youth pastor, Brian Yost. I gave my consent, never suspecting at the time that Brian would soon ask me to go along as their translator. We both began making plans for the missions trip to Mexico the next June.

Also during that winter, I got a call from a man in Christian publishing who wanted me to write something for him. After reading my article in *World Mission People*, he had talked to the magazine's editor about me and then called to ask me to contribute a chapter to a book he was compiling. It was about diversity in the church, and each chapter was being written by someone from a different subgroup in the Body of Christ. My chapter was to be about the contributions that physically challenged believers have to offer the Body. It didn't take long to put my thoughts on paper.

One of the points I tried to make in it was about healing. The issue had caused me a lot of heartache in the past, and I had searched the Scriptures to understand God's perspective on it. I had learned that the Lord does not look down on people with physical problems. In the Old Testament, Moses talked to God about his speech impediment, and God said to him, "Who gave man his mouth? Who makes him deaf or mute? Who gives him sight or makes him blind? Is it not I, the Lord?" (Exodus 4:11) He was essentially saying that he, God, was in control of Moses' limitation.

Similar accounts in the New Testament send the same message. Jesus' disciples once asked him why a particular man had been born blind, and he said, "Neither this man nor his parents sinned, but this happened so that the work of God might be displayed in his life." (John 9:3) And in the case of the Apostle Paul, God refused his request to remove his thorn in the flesh three times. His impairment was actually meant to *prevent* the sin of conceit because of the wonderful things God was doing through him. (2 Cor. 12:7)

When the book's editor read my chapter, he really liked it and made only a few technical changes. The book was published later in the year. I could only hope that my contribution would help people to look at handicaps with greater understanding and acceptance.

The Lord gave me some wonderful women to commute with to SVSU, but I knew it was going to become harder to coordinate our schedules as the field work components of my education required more variable hours of my time. I had to reconsider the possibility of attempting to drive myself. The thought of being behind the wheel of a car was scary since I saw my coordination as still being too poor for the job. My M.R.S. counselor told me they would pay for specialized driver's training and cover the cost of any necessary equipment in a car if I went ahead with it. I determined to be brave and

Starting Over

go for it. After all, the driving instructor would put a stop to it if he saw that I wasn't capable. Then I could say I had at least tried.

My instructor through Challenged Driver Educators (C.D.E.) was a big guy named Larry. He started with an assessment of my physical abilities and determined what types of special equipment I needed. Then he took me to the county fairgrounds a mile from my home for the first lesson. Inside his training car there was a mono-pin mounted on the steering wheel which allowed me to turn it with one hand (the right). To the left of the wheel was a lever which I pushed forward to hit the brake and pulled back to control the accelerator—two jobs with one hand.

Needless to say, I didn't break any speed records during the first few lessons. It was amazing, though, to discover that I could handle the car at low speeds. The task required more gross motor skill than fine motor, and I could see my hands easily in my peripheral field of vision while still watching the road. After only one lesson, we switched to a larger fairgrounds in Bay City. Soon we moved to a nearby residential area, then into city traffic and highway driving. I was increasing my speed and the complexity of the task and handling it well. Finally, we hit the expressway. At 70 miles an hour, it felt like I was moving at Mach speed and the car was going to break apart at any moment. (Funny, it never felt that way when another person was driving.)

I had started the driver's training at the beginning of the winter semester. With five classes plus observations to do at a local high school, I was overloaded and had to suspend the lessons for a while. As soon as the semester was over, I resumed them and got my driver's license in mid-May. Unbelievable!! After fourteen years of depending on others for transportation, I had the privilege to drive myself again. It had not been as hard as I had feared, and I kicked myself (and Denny, too) for not trying sooner.

Now that I was licensed, I needed a vehicle. I had no money to buy one, and M.R.S. could only cover the cost of the special equipment. I was on my own to pay for a car. First, I went with Larry to a local dealership to choose a model. Once I had a price, I went to the bank and asked for a 15-year home mortgage to cover it. I also sent letters to family, friends, and churches that knew me explaining my circumstances and asking if anyone could lend a hand. The donations I received totaled about $3,000. My loan payments were going to be low, but I was also adding insurance, gas, and maintenance costs to a tight budget. Yet, buying a car was the obvious next step in God's plan for me.

My first-ever brand new car was a tan 1999 Taurus with power seats and windows along with other helpful features. Ford's Mobility Motoring paid $1,000 toward my special equipment, and M.R.S. covered the other $3,000. I needed a mono-pin, brake/accelerator lever, and a device called a Chair Topper. The topper would fold and store my manual wheelchair on the roof of the car and require minimal effort on my part to operate. Once the equipment was installed, I would be ready to go.

Becoming a licensed driver again was a monumental event. It was equal to letting go of 24-hour hired help 12 years previously. The impossible had been achieved again. What were my true limits with this handicap, anyway? I wasn't sure but knew I was the only one who could find out. My new long-range goal was to eliminate any barriers to further progress no matter how long it would take to tear each one down.

Starting Over

Year: 2005

Dear Russell,

I want to thank you, son, for your patience and help. There were times when you filled in as my driver to and from the community college. You were also one of my encouragers when I was down. There were many times during the early days of my schooling when I wanted to quit, but you (among others) helped me to keep going. I would have regretted it later if I had surrendered to the hardships and self-pity and dropped out of school. So, thank you!

I wish I could have been less intense back then. I had lived with constant stress for so many years and had such a fear of another trial around every corner. My low self-esteem and victim mentality didn't help either. I think we could have enjoyed your last years at home more if I had been relaxed, self-confident, and easy going. I have improved a lot lately, don't you think?

If there is anything I would want you to learn from our trials, it's this: No matter what happens, God will never leave us or forsake us. When our lives are ripped apart, our bodies afflicted, our hearts broken, and our convictions tested, he is still there. I am not perfect; neither was your dad; neither are you. God loves us anyway. He can bring good out of our mistakes, inadequacies, and even our sins. Never give up, son, no matter what you face in the future. Remember: Life is hard, but God is good. He offers us help and hope and a peace that passes all understanding. Let's take it!

Hugs and kisses,
Mom

Chapter 12

Full Potential

In the late spring of 1999, I was preparing for two major events at the same time—getting my customized car and going to Mexico. Both were very exciting, but I noticed a growing anxiety about the trip. There was a gnawing fear that someone was going to die before Russell and I left the country. I discussed it with Bob, who was still driving down from up north to see me every week after almost four years. We both knew where the fear was coming from: Denny had died right before we had left for Ecuador. I associated a missions trip with the death of a loved one. Talking about it with Bob helped a lot, as always, and I was able to relax.

In preparation for the trip, Brian held several meetings for the team members. There were seven teenagers, including Russell, and three adults—Brian, his wife Laurie, and me. Each teen was asked to write a brief account of his/her relationship with the Lord, and I translated them into Spanish. I also taught them some basic terms in Spanish like "Hello", "Thank you", and "Where's the bathroom?". Laurie taught them some skits that had no dialogues, only actions accompanied by music, but the spiritual message in each one was clear to any observer.

During the same time period, I got my as-yet-unmodified car, and Russell drove me around in it until the day of our departure. Then, on the morning of our flight, we dropped it off at the dealership so they could transport it to Bay City to have the special equipment installed while we were in Mexico.

On June 15, my 42nd birthday, our missions team piled into a van and headed for Detroit Metro. We stopped at a fast-food restaurant along the way so the already-hungry teens could get something to eat, and later we stopped at a rest area. As a result, we were running short on time. Then we got caught in a traffic jam for quite a while. We reached our terminal at the airport with only 20 minutes to spare. We got our baggage out of the van and through the scanner in record time. Then the airline worker at the counter informed us that three of our minors could not board the plane. They only had one parent's signature on their permission forms, not both.

A scramble for a solution led to Laurie's staying behind with the three unhappy teens while the rest of us raced for our gate. Laurie's plan was to contact a local church to take them in for the night, get the needed signatures by fax, and take another flight to Mexico the next day. When the rest of us got to our plane, it was ready to go. To limit our delay time, I told the flight attendants to forget about the aisle-wide wheelchair for me. Russell scooped me up in his arms, whisked me down the aisle to my seat, and plopped me into it before locating his own.

Our flight went straight through to Mexico. After a bumpy descent, we landed in Mexico City, disembarked, and went through Customs. It took a few minutes for me to explain Russell's beef jerky, which must have looked like dynamite on the scanner, and then we were free to meet our contact person. Jorge, the director of the Evangelical Institute of Mexico, and his teenage son helped us load our baggage into their two vehicles, and we traveled to Acopilco (no, that's not Acapulco!) just outside the city where the institute was located.

The male team members were to sleep in two-bed windowless rooms in the dormitory connected to the dining hall while we females had one large, crowded room with six bunk beds in a different building up on the hill. It had once been a garage, but it did have a bathroom. Unfortunately, there was one step up into it and no handi-bar, so the promise of an accessible bathroom had not been valid. During our two weeks in Mexico, we learned that "accessible" doesn't mean barrier-free there; it means the space is large enough for a wheelchair to fit into it. After putting our luggage away, we went to the dining hall for lunch. Before long, some of us sensed something odd.

"This is weird," said one of the girls. "I feel like I'm moving, like I'm still on the plane." Brian felt it, too.

I was too far down the table to hear them. However, I did notice that the trees outside the dining hall were quivering. Suddenly Jorge and another man hurried outside. They came right back, but by then the earthquake was already over. We Michiganders laughed it off, unaware at the moment of the deaths of four people at the epicenter in Puebla to our south.

The next day the other four team members joined us, and our work began. We were taken to various locations, such as churches and parks, where the teens performed their skits and read their testimonies in unrefined Spanish. We also had some games to play with the children, which were used as the ice breakers. All of the teens performed their parts well in the skits and seemed to enjoy their experiences in a different culture.

We had several opportunities for sightseeing. We went to the pyramids built by ancient Indians called Teotihuacan. We went to the huge park in Mexico City where there was a small castle, a zoo, a lake, and lots of vendors selling everything from hand-painted artwork to tacos. In the evenings, our teens played various sports with Jorge's three adolescent children as well as some of the people at the institute. Sometimes they baked cookies or played guitars and sang songs. Strong bonds of friendship developed between the Americans and our Mexican hosts. Since I needed more rest than the others, I missed out on the evening fun. I tried not to be jealous as I lay in bed alone in the women's room on the hill.

During the trip, each person gained a new perspective on some area of life. Laurie had a hard time at first adjusting to the slower pace of living. One girl had a new appreciation for her blessings back home. Almost everyone lost weight since they didn't have frequent access to a refrigerator. Each teen had the opportunity to share his/her testimony in front of a group in addition to being actors. I learned how mentally taxing it can be to translate for almost everyone around me day after day. It was good that Jorge and his son knew a little English. Occasionally, one of our teens would say something memorable. One girl said she would give her right arm to be ambidextrous. (Sorry, sweetie, but that'll never fly.)

At the end of two weeks, we said "good-bye" to our new friends at the institute. A couple of the girls had a hard time leaving. Once we were on the plane, though, everyone's focus shifted to going home as well as meeting their immediate needs. When the flight attendants served lunch, some of our teens boldly asked other passengers for leftover food off their trays. They were so hungry. We flew to Detroit and then traveled on home.

Russell and I listened to the messages left on our answering machine while we were gone and got the shocking news that Ben (Denny and Russell's old hunting partner) had died. We later learned that the cause was a ruptured gall bladder. I couldn't help wondering whether my fear about someone dying before we left had actually been a premonition.

Within days, Russell and I went to Bay City to get my car. Larry, my driving instructor, rode with us on my first trip in the Taurus, which handled somewhat differently than his training car. From then on, I drove without a support person. It took a while to become comfortable driving alone, but the independence was empowering. I relished the freedom to move as fast as everyone else for a change and loved going 70 mph on the expressway with the big guys. My summer course began soon afterward, so I got lots of practice making two trips to Saginaw per week.

Not long after I started driving again, my mother made an interesting comment about my progress.

"We prayed for your healing for years," she said, "but we never imagined anything like this."

For years, we had all looked at wholeness and healing in specific, physical terms. We had not considered that there might be more than one way to be made "whole" again. Becoming a vibrant, productive woman was possible in spite of my physical deficits. I could have dreams and set goals and actually achieve them.

During that summer, a mishap necessitated some home improvements. A dish towel hanging over the oven door handle caught fire one day when I turned the gas oven on. Fortunately, it did not ignite anything else. After burning in place for a moment, it fell on the linoleum floor and soon burned up. The front of the oven was scorched as well as a small section of the flooring. The insurance company gave me enough money to replace the built-in oven and all the linoleum in the house (since it was connected and matched) with a little money to spare. A minor misfortune turned into good fortune.

In the bathroom, I decided to have my built-in cabinet-style bench over the toilet torn out so the whole bathroom floor could be recovered. The friend who dismantled the bench mounted a handi-bar next to the toilet for me. Now I was able to function in my home bathroom in the same way I did in public bathrooms, which helped to strengthen my legs and improve my coordination.

As my third year of college got under way, I was feeling less anxious and less stressed. Although I still had some emotional struggles, the falling dreams had long since ended and I was enjoying life a little more. During that fall, I switched back to the house church. A few of the women in our old congregation had shown concern for my emotional needs, but they were not in a position to offer me much support. I was no longer in need of as much of it and was learning to get by with less than I wanted anyway. Russell (now a senior in high school) and I each had our own cars, making it easier to go to each one's preferred church on Sundays.

With my own set of wheels, I experienced both blessings and burdens. Carpooling was over; there was no need to match my schedule with anyone else's. I didn't have to wait on others to take care of my errand running in town. One of the biggest blessings was being able to go to more of Russell's soccer games. In his first two years in soccer, I was only able to watch two games per season. With my new driving independence, I went to six of them, including the state championship game down state.

The downside of owning a vehicle was the cost and maintenance. My cash reserves were shrinking by the month. Also, I couldn't pump my own gas and therefore had to drive out of my way and past several self-serve stations to get to the full-service ones. I was driving about 360 miles a week just for school and was learning how to drive in even the worst weather conditions.

By January, I knew my finances were in jeopardy. According to my calculations, my current rate of spending was going to deplete all of my savings by June and I would then be unable to make my mortgage payments. Feeling I had no other choice, I listed the house with a realtor I was acquainted with and spent some time looking at handicap apartments closer to the university. Few of them were accessible enough for my needs, and none were available. I had to trust the Lord to work it all out according to his plan.

Emotionally, I lost ground again due to several factors. Being independent in the cold weather was stressful. I often had to drive home from school after dark, sometimes in a snow storm. If the weather was really bad, I would call Russell with my cell phone to keep him posted on my progress on the journey home. Even getting from the car into the building where most of my classes were held was much harder by myself in my manual wheelchair than it had been with a companion to help. In addition, not knowing whether I would have to sell the house and move was very stressful. And then there was Russell's graduation coming up and the prospect of an empty nest.

For years, Russell had planned on joining the military after graduation. He went to the local recruiting office during the winter and was dismayed to learn that his asthma made him ineligible for military service. It had improved significantly in recent years, so the recruiter suggested he see an asthma specialist to get a recommendation. Two trips to Alpena later, Russell had a letter from the specialist saying his mild, intermittent asthma should not keep him out of the military. The recruiter sent it to the appropriate office, but Russell was still turned down.

Also during the winter, he got a call from a man in his church who had his own electrical business. He offered Russell an electrical apprenticeship. Russell didn't know if he would like that kind of work, but the money sounded good. So he accepted the offer, expecting to begin the job right after graduation.

Kathryn had been renting our old house to a young couple for some time. When they moved out in March, she gave Russell permission to move in. He had his Social Security checks to cover most expenses and help with utilities from Grandma. Our 11-year-old dog Donny was his and I didn't want full responsibility for taking care of him, so Russell took Donny with him when he moved out. All of a sudden, I was living alone and my house was very quiet. The resulting loneliness was predictable but difficult. The hardest part was being alone at night. One time I shared my empty-nest emotions with another middle-aged student at the university. At first, she was sympathetic.

"How far away did your son move?" she asked with concern.

"Uh . . . across the street," I answered sheepishly. She laughed at me.

"But it's still hard!" I exclaimed in my own defense. But she was right. I was a fortunate mother to have my son so close by.

I finished the winter semester in late April and had about two weeks off before my spring course began. This was the only year when I took both a spring and summer course. It was necessary to do so if I was going to finish my degree within a five-year period. Even though I had a year's worth of transferable credits from my prior schooling, there were many degree requirements to meet, and the Bilingual Program requirements were adding another year to my education.

Russell graduated from the Baptist school in late May. Among my numerous anxieties had been the fear that something would keep him from finishing high school on time—a half credit short, sickness, whatever. In almost every area of life, I was afraid that a disruption or roadblock would interrupt anything worthwhile we tried to do. It all went back to those years of struggle and the emotional scars they had left. When Russell got his diploma, I breathed a deep sigh of relief. I was also proud that a young man whose family life had been painful in many ways had reached this goal, and I thanked God for it.

By then, Russell's Sundance was on its last leg. We went back to the dealership where we bought it to look at newer vehicles. There was a big red Dodge Ram truck that he wanted, not unlike most 18-year-old males. He had been promised the electrical apprenticeship during the winter but had not yet gotten the call to start. Under pressure to co-sign for the truck, I allowed my ongoing self-doubts and my desire to please him get in the way. I agreed to partner with him on the truck loan against my better judgment. Soon afterward we learned that the apprenticeship offer was being withdrawn because of a lighter work load than the business owner had anticipated, and Russell had to start looking for a different job.

As for my own finances, the house had not been sold by June, my savings were gone, and there was no handicap apartment available anywhere. I was beside myself with anxiety and spoke with Bob about it often. His visits had begun to taper off due to his work load up north and the overall improvement in my situation, but I had frequent contact with him by phone. Despite his encouragement, I felt the weight of my financial need pressing heavily on my shoulders, and I saw the dilemma as mine to solve. One day I called Dr. VonHoff, the director of the Bilingual Program, to tell her I was dropping out of school to look for work and would not be in her class the next day. She encouraged me to take my time in making a decision, but I was sure there was no other way.

The next morning I got up at my usual time and got ready for the day, not knowing what I should do with it. During my prayer time, however, I felt a renewed determination surge through me regarding my finances. The Lord seemed to be saying to me, "Your job is to go to school. Let me handle the finances." I went to class after all, and Dr. VonHoff told me I had made her day. I told two of my Latina women friends, Daisy and Vicki, who were in the class with me, about my struggle. They were shocked.

"This isn't the Mae Jean we know!" they said. "You're a woman of faith; this isn't like you."

They promised to pray for me and to call their believing friends to ask them to pray for me, too. They said I should call all my friends and ask them to pray as well. Daisy and Vicki gave me encouragement while at the same time pricking my conscience. I didn't like being a person who would exercise great faith in one area and quake with fear in another. It was hard on me and a poor testimony to others.

About a week later, the realtor came by the house and asked how I was doing. When I told her my savings were gone, she offered to lend me as much as I needed to get me by until the house sold. Her offer was a Godsend. In September, her son and his wife bought it as an investment. I had not been able to find another place to live, but they were willing to rent the house to me until my circumstances changed.

After paying off the mortgage, I used some of my equity to buy a computer to help me with school work, a front-loading washer, and some other helpful items for my home. I put a small amount of the money into the stock market, which I had never invested in before, but the bulk of it went into savings. I didn't know when or whether I would move but was deeply grateful to the Lord for letting me stay in my special house.

My fourth year of college went by without any major changes in my life. Despite my academic success, I approached each semester as a whole new game. I worked just as hard, knowing my past success had not come without significant effort. There were many times when I wanted my involvement at SVSU to go beyond academics. I wanted to attend the plays, recitals, football games, etc. Unfortunately, I lived too far away and had little free time. I did develop some good friendships with my classmates and knew they were enriching my life. I remained cautious, however, about forming long-term emotional bonds with them. When we graduated, we were all going our separate ways, and I still did not want to face any painful separations.

In some ways, my relationship with Wes was still causing emotional pain. He and Alta had come back from China, and I hoped they would visit me or at least call me once in a while. But their lives had been changing, too. When I first met them, their two sons were not yet married. Since then, two daughters-in-law and four grandchildren had been added to their close-knit family. Wes and Alta had less time now to spend with their friends. Generally, I would see them if they came to my area to visit all their local friends or if I drove up north. The hardest part was not understanding why they didn't at least call me. Wes was one of the few people who understood what I had been through and was still going through as a middle-aged handicapped widow.

On several occasions, I tried talking to Wes about it by phone, but it didn't help. In fact, it made matters worse. One day he finally admitted that he felt like he had to walk on eggs when talking to me. In my effort to change the relationship, I was only straining it and making him uncomfortable. I had to learn to accept the relationship as it was, not as I wanted it to be.

Over the previous year or two, I had learned that it was better to avoid people when I needed something they couldn't or wouldn't give me than to create a strain in the relationship by pressing for it. So I adopted the same approach with Wes. When I was hurting the most, I stayed away from church services and didn't initiate contact with anyone but Bob. He still came to see me occasionally when his schedule allowed him to, and he encouraged me to call whenever I needed to talk. His friendship meant so much to me.

When my fourth year of college ended in the spring of 2001, I had just five courses left before my student teaching. The final requirement for the Bilingual Program was a six-week field project working in a migrant summer school program. The closest one to my house was 40 minutes away. In late June, I started the project assuming I would work with secondary students, but there were only three high school students initially in attendance. There was a significant need, however, for helpers in the lower grades, so I was assigned to work with the three- to eight-year-old group throughout the program.

During that summer, I did some soul searching because of my never-ending struggle with self-esteem. It had improved some since Denny's death, but there was no justification for the degree of my ongoing negative self-criticism. God had blessed me so much. How could I go on doubting my worth in his sight? Sometimes I was my own worst enemy, being much harder on myself than I would have been on another person. One day it occurred to me that it was actually a sin to love myself less than the Father loved me. It was an epiphany.

From then on, I tried to live by the baby girl dream God had given me years earlier. I worked at being my own best friend, changing my self-talk from negative to positive. Life became much more enjoyable, and my relationships improved. I could initiate contact with others, particularly Wes and Alta, more frequently because I was less in need of their affirmation and better equipped to give in small ways.

I remembered a statement Rose had shared with me once from her counseling with Wes. For people like us, Wes said there were layers of emotional issues to peel back like the layers of an onion. Often it was necessary to peel them off one at a time. During my counseling with him and Bob, I had removed several layers related to my handicap, marriage, and beliefs. During the year of Denny's cancer, new layers were added as rapidly as old ones were removed. But my life had changed since then. I was making progress in all areas of life, more rapidly in some than in others.

One of the areas of very slow change had been my outlook on my life's circumstances. I had felt like a victim for years—first because of the medical mistake, then the abuse, and then the events that left me a widow. But in the process of becoming a more independent and productive person, the victim mentality had faded away. I recognized that it only slowed me down whenever I gave in to self-pity or brooding over life's hardships. Enough time had been wasted; I didn't want to rob myself of the good things I was capable of by dwelling on the negative.

As the fall semester of 2001 got under way, I knew these were my last classes and the frequent trips to Saginaw would end in December. The possibility of doing my student teaching at a local high school during the winter semester was almost 100 percent. On the morning of September 11, I did my homework for my class later in the day without taking any breaks to watch TV or listen to the radio. Since the class met from 4:00 to 7:00 p.m., I was going to miss the evening news and so decided to watch the local news at noon. I was completely unaware of the terrorist attacks and WTC towers collapse which had occurred while I studied. When I turned the TV on, I learned about all of it at once and was in total shock.

I reacted in two ways. First, I was as horrified as everyone else by what had taken place and believed that the world would never be the same again. Second, all my fears of another tragedy ripping my life apart came rushing back. Initially, I took the attacks very personally. *This is it, the next battle*, I thought as my heart pounded. It took weeks to work through my emotions. The new war on terrorism was only my war to the extent that it was every American's war. The terrorist attacks were not a personal attack on me, nor did they alter my daily life. I did not live in the targeted places, no one I knew lived there, I didn't fly often, and my son could not go to war because of his asthma.

During the winter semester, I did my student teaching at a high school about 12 miles from my house. My host teacher, Linda, taught both of the languages I had studied and was a 27-year veteran. After observing for about two weeks, I took over the two Spanish I classes. A couple weeks later, I added the Spanish II section. I was able to handle the work fairly well, but there was a growing problem. I was pushing myself to keep up with the full-time work hours and with meals and housework at home. In my Christmas letter to family and friends, I had said I would appreciate any practical help they could give me during student teaching, but no help came. Although Rose wanted to provide some meals, the circumstances of her life made it too hard for her to carry through on her intentions.

An unrelated problem also affected my work. As March 9 and 15 (Denny's birth and death dates) drew closer, I thought I would handle the emotions okay since this was now the fifth anniversary of his death. When those dates actually arrived, however, I was overcome with emotion once again. I started breaking down at school and taking whole or partial days off.

Linda was understanding but concerned for me. Something needed to change and fast, or my student teaching was going to end in failure.

Several times over the years I had considered taking an antidepressant. One time I got samples from my doctor but then changed my mind. I never felt at peace with using a drug to solve my emotional problems. With nearly five years of hard work now in jeopardy, I went to the doctor, got some more samples, and began taking them. Just days later our spring break started, and I hoped to be emotionally stable by the time it was over. Soon I became noticeably more fatigued, assumed it was the drug, and stopped taking it. If I was going to succeed in student teaching, it would be on my own.

At a teacher inservice held just prior to spring break, I saw an old friend named Mary Aliene who was teaching in the elementary school. We had met as girls attending the same church with our families. We had had little contact since becoming adults but had seen each other a couple of times at SVSU. She had also gotten her teaching degree as a middle-aged single mother. When I told her of my struggle to keep up with my schedule, she offered to bring in meals and do anything else that would be helpful. She was the answer to my prayers.

When we returned to school, there were only three weeks left in my student teaching. The painful anniversary was behind me, I had rested up during my time off, and Mary Aliene was bringing me several meals per week. Not only that, each time she came to the house she would spend time encouraging me and praying with me. It made all the difference in the world. Linda saw a dramatic change for the better in me. I began teaching the French II class, and in the last week I took on the fifth and final class, French I, thus giving me a full teaching load. I finished the 14-week project with a tremendous sense of accomplishment.

There were two special events to attend at the university as I completed my degree. One was for the students majoring in education and their host teachers. The other was the Honors Convocation, which I chose to attend in place of the commencement because it was much smaller and more personal. My parents and Russell were able to be there with me. My final GPA was 3.99. With my educational goal achieved, I recalled Wes' comment years before about having high hopes for me. I called him and asked if this was what he had envisioned for me back then. His reply? Yes, and more!

For the next month, I was so happy and peaceful I slept like a baby. I did a little substitute teaching and earned my first paychecks since Russell's birth. There was no summer class to attend; I was all done! My new focus was on finding a job. I made some contacts but didn't get any calls for work through most of the summer. I used the time off to get out a little more. I even drove 300 miles to Elkhart, Indiana, to go to my first rodeo with my sister Pam and her children. It was the farthest I had ever driven alone in my entire life, proof positive that I was becoming a more daring and adventurous person.

In August, I got a few job calls and had two interviews, both down state. I remained open to the possibility of moving, though I was desperately hoping for a local job. But as the schools opened for the 2002-2003 academic year, I had no job and was very disappointed. Yet, I knew God was not asleep or on vacation. He would give me something to do for the next 12 months.

Many people who had read my first book had asked me over the years when I was going to write another one. The same question had come up again during the summer. My answer was always the same: I couldn't write until God gave me the time and the inspiration. What most people were not told was that I didn't want to relive the pain of the past nor face the criticism I anticipated if I shared the negative side of my marriage to a man who had been dearly loved by many. Although I had sensed for a long time that God would one day require the writing of a second book, I pleaded with him not to make me do it.

Suddenly, I found myself with plenty of time to write, but I still needed something from the Lord to give me the courage to begin. On praying about it, an inner voice said, "Haven't you come far enough by now to deal with the criticism? If you do what God wants, you don't need anybody's approval." And so I began to write.

Days later I got a call for a part-time job at a high school more than 30 miles away. It involved teaching Spanish for only one class period on block scheduling, which meant going to the school every other day for about two hours. In addition to a small salary, I was offered mileage reimbursement. Needless to say, I took the job. Although it didn't provide enough income to buy the house back, it significantly slowed the depletion of my remaining savings.

Most importantly, it left me time for writing. In the process of recounting the painful experiences which had been emotionally devastating to me, I gained new clarity and insight on many issues and events. I discovered that I could face the pain of the past and benefit from it. Writing about it left me with a feeling of closure and release from the past. By the time I was finished with the bulk of the manuscript, I was thanking God for making me write it!

The following summer, I learned that Linda, my host teacher during student teaching, had retired. I applied for her position and was hired for the 2003-2004 school year. That first full year of teaching was exhausting. There was so much to learn and adjust to—not just professionally but also physically. In addition, time was given to securing a mortgage to buy the house back and to helping my parents whose health issues (especially Mom's) became much more serious and potentially life threatening. But I made it through and was told by my mentor teacher that I had accomplished a lot in spite of all the hardships.

My second year has been easier and more meaningful. From the start, I have felt much more confident and organized. In the fall, I was able to take my Spanish II students to SVSU for Foreign Language Day, and they really enjoyed it. I see the potential for next year to be even better as I continue to gain experience and confidence.

Today Russell and I are doing well. He still lives in our old house on the farm. He has worked several low-paying and/or short-term jobs to get by with his main job being in construction during the warm-weather months. Two summers ago he opened a vegetable stand, which earns him significant extra cash during July and August. Old Donny dog is no longer with us, but his place in the family has been filled by Nicki, a black lab. Like his father, Russell has been a successful hunter, beginning with an eight-point buck he shot when he was 16. He also has an interest in amateur boxing and is making a second attempt to get into the military.

As for me, my life is more normal now than it has been since becoming handicapped 20 years ago. I rarely feel anxious about the possibility of more hardship and heartache to come. Instead, I look forward with anticipation to the continual unfolding of God's plan for the rest of my life. For a long time I thought that I had been sentenced to a life of pain and would never be truly happy again this side of heaven. I was so wrong!

Have I reached my full potential yet? Almost. I have tried doing more leg exercises and using a walker, but it takes about ten minutes to walk ten feet and I dare not look away from my legs or remove even one hand from the walker to use it for something else. So I doubt that my physical abilities are going to increase. Emotionally, there are still a few lingering issues to work on. I have known for some time that negative emotions slow me down physically. If I can overcome them, I will feel even better on the inside and be more productive on the outside. Then I will probably need less rest, which will give me more time for the things I want to do.

As I have worked on updating this writing project for the last time before publication, I have been amazed by my own experiences. Reading about the physical trauma sent shudders through me; I can hardly believe I survived. Later, the marriage problems and cancer were as hard to recover from as the nerve damage. My own resiliency astounds me, but I know it is the result of God's power to strengthen the weak when their own strength is gone. He is an awesome God! Where do I go from here? Anywhere he leads me.

Year: 2005

Dear Bob,

From the time you took over the counseling in 1994 until today, you've been the first person I call when I need advice or just a listening ear. Even though our contact is strictly by phone now, you are still my best friend, my safest place to fall. You had no idea what you were getting yourself into by volunteering to work with us, did you? Of course, God knew. He could see into the future and knew I was going to need someone who was steady when I was unsteady. He knew about the trials and the triumphs that lay ahead and the kind of person I needed to walk through it with me.

One of the things I have really appreciated about both you and Wes is that you showed compassion without pitying me. Have you ever seen the old movie *The Miracle Worker*? I like the part where Annie Sullivan, the teacher, is looking at blind, deaf Helen and says, "No pity. I won't have it." Pity lacks hope and expects little or nothing. It keeps an afflicted person down and helpless. Compassion, on the other hand, connects and then helps in a productive way. It seeks to strengthen and enable until there is no temptation to pity.

Thank you for allowing God to use you as my counselor, friend, and coach. I don't think it was a coincidence that God picked a part-time football coach to support me. Thanks for helping me get back into the game of life!

With great love,
Mae Jean

To contact the author of

OUT OF THE Tempest

Mae Jean Mason
1779 E. M-55
Prescott, MI 48756
(989) 345-5043
mjmason@m33access.com